B. G. A. Moynihan

On retro-peritoneal Hernia

Being the 'Arris and Gale' Lectures

B. G. A. Moynihan

On retro-peritoneal Hernia
Being the 'Arris and Gale' Lectures

ISBN/EAN: 9783337162863

Printed in Europe, USA, Canada, Australia, Japan

Cover: Foto ©ninafisch / pixelio.de

More available books at **www.hansebooks.com**

ON

RETRO-PERITONEAL HERNIA.

BEING

The 'Arris and Gale' Lectures

ON

'THE ANATOMY AND SURGERY OF THE PERITONEAL FOSSÆ,'

DELIVERED AT THE

Royal College of Surgeons of England.

BY

B. G. A. MOYNIHAN, M.S. (Lond.), F.R.C.S. (Eng.), etc.,
ASSISTANT SURGEON LEEDS GENERAL INFIRMARY.

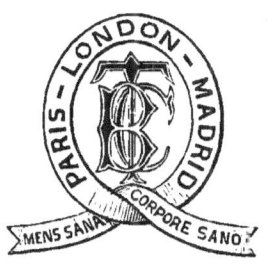

LONDON:
BAILLIÈRE, TINDALL AND COX,
20 & 21, KING WILLIAM STREET, STRAND.
[PARIS AND MADRID.]
1899.
[All rights reserved.]

TO

T. R. JESSOP,

CONSULTING SURGEON TO THE LEEDS GENERAL INFIRMARY, MEMBER OF
THE COUNCIL, ROYAL COLLEGE OF SURGEONS OF ENGLAND,

TO WHOSE TEACHING AND EXAMPLE

I OWE MORE THAN ANY WORDS OF MINE CAN

ADEQUATELY EXPRESS,

I AFFECTIONATELY DEDICATE THIS BOOK.

PREFACE.

This volume contains the lectures which, as 'Arris and Gale' lecturer, I had the honour of delivering at the Royal College of Surgeons in February and March of this year.

The subject of retro-peritoneal hernia has received less than adequate attention from English surgeons in the past. The condition is not an exceptionally rare one, for, in addition to the cases recorded, I have found a few undescribed specimens in the London museums. The photographs of all the specimens that exist in the museums of England and Scotland, so far as I have been able to ascertain, are placed at the end of the book.

My attention was first drawn to the subject by a case which occurred at the Leeds General Infirmary some years ago. Several of those present at the post-mortem examination of this case attempted an explanation of the peritoneal conditions which existed. The discussion interested me, and ever since I have made, both in the dissecting-room and, when opportunity occurred, in the post-mortem-room, a long series of observations. The result has been that I have been able to describe from actual, prolonged, and repeated observation, a large number of peritoneal fossæ, some of which had either escaped recognition altogether, or early descriptions of them had been lost sight of. In every case where a vestige of old peritonitis has been present, I have omitted to make any record.

Soon after my observations were commenced, it became apparent to me that the conditions of the fossæ varied considerably with the age of the patient. In the young, the fossæ and their determining folds were much more clearly and accurately defined. In later years changes were induced by traction effects, the deposit of fat, and so forth. I therefore made a point of examining a large number of fœtuses. Owing to the kindness of many medical friends, notably Drs. Woodcock, Waite, Ellison, and Knowles, I have had an abundant supply of material. To the fœtal, as contrasted with the adult, fossæ I have made frequent allusion.

The drawings are in some cases original. Some are copied from Jonnesco, some from Brösike. All of them, whether copies or original, have been done for me by Mr. J. W. Haigh. For the photographs of the specimens in the London museums I am indebted to Mr. Godart, of Fleet Street.

I wish to express my thanks to the curators of the St. Bartholomew's, St. Thomas's, Guy's, and St. Mary's museums, and to the authorities of the Royal College of Surgeons, for their courteous permission to view and photograph their specimens.

For two very beautiful examples of duodenal hernia, one of the 'right' variety and one of the 'left,' I am indebted to my friend and colleague, Dr. T. Wardrop Griffith.

B. G. A. M.

LEEDS.

TABLE OF CONTENTS.

CHAPTER I.

PAGE

THE DEVELOPMENT OF THE INTESTINAL CANAL AND PERITONEUM - - - - - 9

CHAPTER II.

THE DUODENAL FOLDS AND FOSSÆ - - - 19
   HISTORY OF THE VARIOUS FOSSÆ FOUND IN THE NEIGHBOURHOOD OF THE DUODENO-JEJUNAL FLEXURE - - - - - 19
   DESCRIPTION OF THE FOLDS AND FOSSÆ - - 25
      1. THE SUPERIOR DUODENAL FOSSA - - 25
      2. THE INFERIOR DUODENAL FOSSA - - 27
      3. THE POSTERIOR DUODENAL FOSSA - - 28
      4. THE DUODENAL-JEJUNAL FOSSA - - 29
      5. THE INTER-MESOCOLIC FOSSA - - 31
      6. THE INFRA-DUODENAL FOSSA - - 32
      7. THE PARA-DUODENAL FOSSA - - - 33
      8. THE MESENTERICO-PARIETAL FOSSA, OR FOSSA OF WALDEYER - - - - - 36
      9. THE PARA-JEJUNAL FOSSA - - - 36
   ORIGIN OF THE FOLDS AND FOSSÆ - - - 40
   DUODENAL HERNIA - - - - - 42
      LEFT DUODENAL HERNIA - - - - 43
         POINT OF ORIGIN - - - - 43
         CONDITIONS PREDISPOSING TO THE HERNIA - 46
         THE NECK OF THE SAC - - - 46
         THE SIZE OF THE HERNIA - - - 50
         HISTORY - - - - - 54
      RIGHT DUODENAL HERNIA - - - - 56
         POINT OF ORIGIN - - - - 56
         CONDITIONS PREDISPOSING TO THE HERNIA - 58
         THE NECK OF THE SAC, ETC. - - 59
         ENUMERATION OF CASES - - - 64
   PERIOD OF ONSET OF DUODENAL HERNIA - - 65
   DIAGNOSIS - - - - - - 66
      PHYSICAL SIGNS - - - - - 67
   TREATMENT - - - - - - 70

CHAPTER III.

THE PERITONEAL FOLDS AND POUCHES IN THE NEIGHBOURHOOD OF THE CÆCUM AND VERMIFORM APPENDIX - 71

   HISTORY OF THE CÆCAL FOSSÆ - . . . 72
   THE ILEO-COLIC ARTERY AND ITS BRANCHES - . 74
   DESCRIPTION OF THE PRIMARY FOLDS AND FOSSÆ - 77
      THE ANTERIOR VASCULAR OR ILEO-COLIC FOLD - 77
      THE ANTERIOR VASCULAR OR ILEO-COLIC FOSSA - 79
      THE ACCESSORY ANTERIOR VASCULAR FOSSA - 80
      THE POSTERIOR VASCULAR FOLD—MESO-APPENDIX - 80
      THE INTERMEDIATE OR ILEO-APPENDICULAR FOLD - 82
      THE ILEO-APPENDICULAR FOSSA - . . 84
      THE FOSSA OF HARTMANN - . . . 85
      THE RETRO-COLIC, RETRO-CÆCAL, FOSSA - 87
      THE PARIETO-COLIC FOLD - . . . 88
      THE MESENTERICO-PARIETAL FOLD - . 88
      THE FOSSA ILIACO-SUBFASCIALIS—FOSSA OF BIESIADECKI - 90
   GENESIS OF THE FOLDS AND FOSSÆ - . . 90
   PERICÆCAL HERNIA - 96
      ILEO-APPENDICULAR HERNIA - . . 96
   HERNIA INTO THE FOSSA OF HARTMANN - . 101
   HERNIA INTO THE RETRO-COLIC FOSSA - . 102
   RETRO-PERITONEAL HERNIA OF THE VERMIFORM PROCESS 108
   HERNIA INTO THE FOSSA OF BIESIADECKI - . 110

CHAPTER IV.

THE INTERSIGMOID FOSSA 112

   HISTORY 112
   DESCRIPTION OF THE FOSSA . . . 114
   GENESIS OF THE FOSSA 116
   HERNIA INTO THE INTERSIGMOID FOSSA . 119

CHAPTER V.

THE FORAMEN OF WINSLOW 127

   ANATOMY - 127
   HERNIA INTO THE FORAMEN . . . 127
      SYMPTOMS - 140
      TREATMENT - 140

ALPHABETICAL LIST OF REFERENCES . . 142

DESCRIPTION OF THE PLATES 151

ON
RETRO-PERITONEAL HERNIA.

CHAPTER I.

THE DEVELOPMENT OF THE INTESTINAL CANAL AND PERITONEUM.

THE intestinal canal, at the beginning of the fourth week of intra-uterine life, consists of an almost straight tube, attached throughout its whole length by a dorsal or posterior fold of peritoneum to the middle line of the body (Fig. 1). This fold is the primitive mesentery. In that portion of the canal which afterwards develops into the stomach is seen a dorsal bulging, which represents the greater curvature of that organ. It is to this curvature, therefore, that the primitive mesentery is attached. From the anterior (or ventral) portion of the stomach, and the beginning of the duodenum, a second fold of peritoneum runs forward to be fixed into the anterior abdominal wall. In this fold, the small omentum, the liver is showing early signs of development.

By the sixth week the intestinal tract can be seen to consist of three segments, each of which is the territory of a special artery by which it is supplied (Fig. 2, *a, b, c*).

The first segment consists of the stomach and duodenum, attached by the mesentery containing the cœliac axis. This primitive mesentery is known as the mesogaster, or, more properly, as the mesogastrioduodenum. The stomach is placed, with its lesser curvature, in front and to the right, its greater curvature to the left and behind; the fundus is above, and the pylorus below, nearly in the middle line. The surfaces look laterally, the left being slightly inclined to the front. At the junction of the pylorus with the duodenum is a curve, the convexity of which is to the front and right. In the mesentery of the concavity of this curve lies the head of the pancreas, the body and tail of which extend to the left, upwards, and backwards in the mesogaster. Above the tail of the pancreas, also in the mesogaster, the spleen lies. The distal end of the duodenum, where later the flexura duodeno-

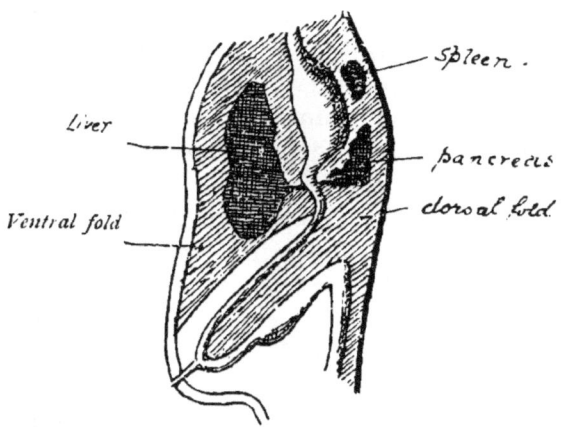

FIG. 1.—ANTERO-POSTERIOR SECTION OF THE TRUNK OF AN EARLY EMBRYO. (HERTWIG.)

jejunalis is found, lies in the median plane of the body, and possesses no mesentery. It is here at a very early period fixed to the posterior abdominal wall, and at this point the duodenum forms, with the first portion of the jejunum, a curve whose concavity is forward.

The second segment of the intestinal canal extends from the flexura duodeno-jejunalis in a long loop (the umbilical loop of Toldt) to the umbilicus, and back to the posterior abdominal wall. This loop consists of a proximal portion, a curvature and a distal portion. The two limbs of the loop run almost parallel with one another, and are united by a long narrow mesentery containing the superior mesenteric artery. In an early stage, the proximal limit of the loop lies more to the right, and this results in the whole umbilical loop with its mesentery lying in a plane which tends to the horizontal. The loop corresponds to the jejunum, ileum, cæcum, ascending and transverse colon. The first indication of the appearance of the cæcum is a slight bulging on the wall of the canal somewhere near the mid-point of the distal section of the loop. The portion of the umbilical loop before the

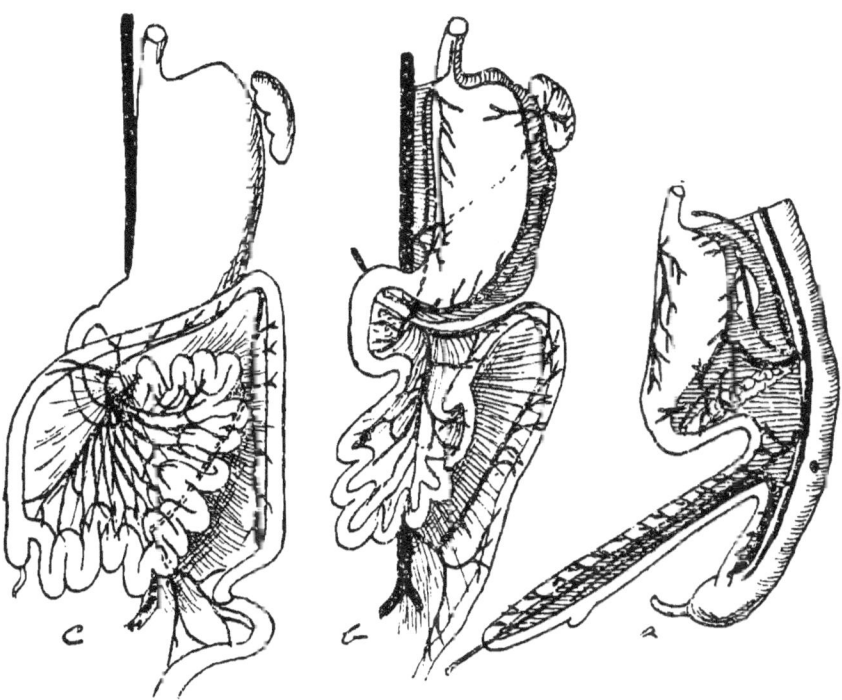

FIG. 2.—*a, b, c*, SUBSEQUENT DEVELOPMENTS IN THE INTESTINAL CANAL, SHOWING THE ARTERIES SUPPLIED TO EACH SEGMENT. (TOLDT.)

point where the cæcum develops is relatively larger than the portion beyond. The termination of the loop is at a rather acute bend, subsequently the splenic flexure of the colon.

At this point begins the third segment of the intestinal tract, which extends from the splenic flexure downwards, and includes the descending colon, sigmoid (omega) loop, and rectum. It has a short, narrow mesentery, within which lies the inferior mesenteric artery.

The subsequent developments of the various sections of the canal are of great importance.

SUBSEQUENT DEVELOPMENT OF THE ABDOMINAL ORGANS.

The subsequent alterations in the relative positions and conditions of the various organs, including the intestine, large and small, are due in great measure to the disproportionate increase in growth of these organs. As this increase has to be confined within the restricted limit of the abdominal cavity, it results that each organ has necessarily some influence on the relative growth and subsequent position of every other organ, and that every organ must of necessity adapt itself to its surroundings.

The first change is in the position and size of the stomach (Fig. 2, *b*, *c*), which undergoes an increase in size, developing still more its greater curvature. There is also now a rotation of this organ in such manner that the left surface becomes anterior, and its right posterior. Such twisting can alone be accomplished by a simultaneous lengthening of the mesentery, and we find consequently that the mesogaster undergoes a very marked increase, leading, in fact, to the formation of a fold or curtain, subsequently the great omentum, which presents, like the stomach, an anterior and a posterior surface. In the third month this bulging is already easily recognisable. Throughout its whole extent, this hanging reduplication of peritoneum is everywhere free of adhesions, and extends from the greater curvature of the stomach to its dorsal median attachment near the pancreas and the spleen.

Synchronous with this alteration in the size and position of the stomach, there occurs a change in the duodenum. There we find that a curve is formed whose convexity is behind and to the right, the upper and lower ends of the curve remaining in the middle line relatively stationary. The result is that the right aspect of the duodenum, and its close neighbour, the head of the pancreas, become more and more closely applied to the hinder wall of the abdomen in its right half.

The most marked alteration and increase occurs simultaneously in the umbilical loop of Toldt (Fig. 2, *b*, *c*). The first sign of this is a relatively large increase in its proximal limb, in the apex, and in the distal segment as far as the cæcum. Much more slowly the large intestine portion of the loop develops. The result is that the swiftly increasing and enlarging coils of small intestine occupying the right and lower portion of the abdomen, and the cæcum and the large intestine, are cramped in the upper and left regions. The cæcum itself lies then above the umbilicus, and at or near the median line of the body. The mesentery of all this loop is at the same time undergoing a correspondingly large increase, changing, as Toldt very aptly and correctly expresses it, from a closed to an open fan. This is the more correct, seeing that it is only the ventral portion of it that is largely increased. The dorsal attachment, containing the root-trunk of the superior mesenteric artery, is still narrow, and fixed to the posterior abdominal wall in an almost horizontal line

Meanwhile, an enormous enlargement of the liver is noticeable, and the organ seems to occupy almost the whole of the upper part of the abdominal cavity.

The alterations in growth of the third intestinal segment are relatively unimportant, and consist merely in an elongation and enlargement of the gut. The mesentery, however, is largely increased, and, as the right side of the abdominal cavity is filled with small intestines, this segment is pushed well over to the left side. Rather early on, the position of the sigmoid flexure is marked by a local increase of growth.

It is at this stage of the development of the abdominal organs that we first meet with the conditions which were first described by Toldt as 'physiological adhesions.' It was observed that under certain conditions, which even yet are by no means thoroughly understood or appreciated, but which are based upon three chief factors, there occurred a growing together of contiguous or adjacent portions of organs, gut, or abdominal wall, covered by peritoneum. The factors in producing these conditions—factors which in most cases would seem to be essential—are:

    1. The close approximation of the peritoneal surfaces.
    2. The absence of movement in areas so placed; or,
    3. The occurrence of a violent rubbing together, and consequent denudation of surfaces of peritoneum which are closely applied to each other.

Conditions 2 and 3 seem doubtless contradictory; but it is hard to find a satisfactory explanation of all cases. Thus, the opposing areas of peritoneum on the upper surface of the liver and the diaphragm are constantly in apposition, and are but little movable; yet they practically never unite. The opposing surfaces of the layer of the great omentum are always in contact, and there is always some movement, not amounting to violent friction, between them; yet they practically always unite.

The reasons, therefore, for such agglutination are still obscure, and the proffering of these points as a tentative explanation is the most that can at present be done to clear the matter up.

At points where this process of physiological adhesion is about to occur, we notice either a dimming in the clearness of the peritoneum, a local turbidity, or an actual thickening of the opposed surfaces. On gently separating such areas, where the fusion has not yet been completed, there are to be seen fine strands of tissue, forming a rough network, extending between the two. When adhesion is completed, there is usually seen a white line, or a more or less broad band of thickening, which Toldt designates as a 'fusion line.'

That such changes did occur, and that adhesions, and blendings, and bindings together were normal in the peritoneal processes, had, of course, long been a matter of universal knowledge. Haller and Meckel first demonstrated such an event in the case of the great omentum and the transverse colon. Treitz speaks of such thickenings and adhesion of the peritoneum, but refers them to fœtal peritonitis. He also mentions the subdivision of the fossa duodeno-jejunalis by bands or serous folds, which are now looked upon as 'physiological adhesions.'

Reference to similar conditions in the mesocolon and in the formation of the ligamentum phrenico-lienale and phrenico-colicum was made by Langer. Waldeyer also was acquainted with such manifestations; but he, and indeed all those I have named, looked upon them either as the remnants of a fœtal peritonitis, or as unexplained and insignificant episodes. It is to Toldt that we are indebted for the view that such adhesions are normal, are physiological, and are essential to the regular and proportionate development of the peritoneum, and to the ultimate peculiar and intrinsic position occupied by each organ.

The first occurrence of this process is noticed in connection with the peritoneum in relation to the pancreas. This organ lies at first between two parallel surfaces of peritoneum; but, as it follows the duodenum in its migration, the posterior layer becomes opposed to, and ultimately fused with, the parietal peritoneum of the posterior abdominal wall.

An important blending similar to this occurs in connection with the mesially-placed portion of the large intestine, developed from the distal limb of the umbilical loop with the original left and ultimate anterior wall of the descending portion of the duodenum. The point of fusion later becomes the hepatic flexure of the colon, and divides therefore the large intestine, developed from this segment of the loop into the cæcum and ascending colon on the one hand, and the transverse colon on the other. It is, according to Brösike, this adhesion between the hepatic flexure and the left side of the duodenum which, in the bending of the latter to the right, gives the original impulse to the movement of the cæcum and ascending colon to the right side of the abdomen. Subsequent to this fusion there follows also a blending of the mesentery of the transverse colon with that portion of the peritoneum (originally left, now anterior) covering the duodenum and the pancreas.

As the duodenum in its movement to the right bends further and further over, its posterior covering of peritoneum comes into contact, precisely as in the case of the pancreas, with the posterior parietal peritoneum, and becomes, of course, amalgamated with that. The first portion of the duodenum to meet with the parietal peritoneum is the terminal segment, and it is here that the union of opposed peritoneal surfaces first occurs. From here the fusion spreads upwards along the head of the pancreas and the descending portion of the duodenum.

At the completion of the development and fixing of the transverse mesocolon there occurs its adhesion to the great omentum in the manner first described by Haller and Meckel.

To the left this extends into the phreno-colic ligament, and to the right into the hepato-colic.

The cæcum meanwhile has changed its position from the middle line of the body just below the liver to the right iliac fossa by travelling at first to the right, and then almost vertically downwards. Subsequent to, and in consequence of, that manœuvre, there occurs a physiological fusion of the mesocolon to the posterior parietal peritoneum of the lower portion of the duodenal ring and the head of the pancreas, and later of the right kidney. On the anterior surface of the duodenum and the head of the pancreas, this fusion extends along a line drawn from the hepatic to the duodenal flexure— a line which corresponds to the insertion of the transverse mesocolon on the posterior abdominal wall. The lateral fusion on the right posterior abdominal wall is posterior to the ascending colon.

The fusion of the fan-shaped portion of mesentery with the parietal peritoneum is along an oblique line extending from the flexura duodeno-jejunalis to the iliac fossa, and thus is formed the permanent line of attachment of the mesentery of the small intestine.

The final physiological fusion takes place between the descending mesocolon and the left posterior parietal peritoneum.

It had been long taught by Treitz, Luschka, Hyrtl, and Waldeyer, that the disappearance of the descending mesocolon was due to its outspreading, owing to the continued growth of the posterior abdominal wall, and the increase in size of the kidney in such manner that the mesocolon was 'used up,' so to speak, in the formation of parietal peritoneum. It was, however, shown by Langer, and later and more completely by Toldt, that the process was one of fusion.

When the descending colon is, by the growth of the small intestines, pushed over to the left, its mesentery still retains its attachment at or near the middle line of the body. The posterior or left layer of the descending colon comes therefore in apposition to the posterior parietal peritoneum, and it is here that the amalgamation of the layers takes place. This fusion is typical of the rest. The union is at first loose, and easily torn through; on drawing the layers apart, it can be seen that the blending occurs at first by means of fine strands of thin, easily-torn tissue, forming a loose, irregular network. This later disappears when the two layers are indissolubly united. This process will be referred to subsequently, when the genesis of the intersigmoid fossa is discussed.

The above description applies to the typical cases. It is, of course, not infrequent to find some modification in one or other site, or of greater or less extent; but any variation so existing must, as Toldt insists, be looked upon as abnormal.

It is possible, also, that this process of physiological agglutination may occur after birth during the early months of extra-uterine life. The most obvious example of this takes place in the case of the opposing layer of the great omentum, the cavity in which becomes thereby to a greater or less extent obliterated.

According to Toldt, a similar fusion may occur in the upper and lower portions of the freely-hanging small intestine. There results, then, an adhesion of the upper few inches of the jejunum, or the lower few inches of the ileum, to the posterior abdominal wall. The existence of this fusion of the jejunum plays possibly a most important, and till very recently overlooked, part in the predisposition to one form of duodenal hernia. This point will receive a closer attention subsequently.

The anomalies of position of the vermiform appendix are numerous. In some of its irregular sites it may become, by a similar process, fixed down to the peritoneum, sometimes of the cæcum, sometimes of the mesentery, sometimes of the posterior abdominal wall. Such adhesions, and, in fact, many of those already enumerated, have been from time to time, and by numerous observers, considered and described as results of a fœtal or infantile peritonitis. As such, however, they can hardly be reckoned, when we take into account the total absence of any similar irregularities elsewhere in the peritoneum. A fœtal peritonitis would lead, presumably, if not certainly, to a more intense and widespread agglutination of opposing surfaces, and to the obvious and extensive building up of scar masses. In the slighter cases a differential diagnosis might be difficult; but the observation of a large number of cases has, since the day when Toldt first fixed our attention on the subject, left little doubt as to the physiological, rather than the pathological, causation of such variations of the appendix as I have referred to. In the case of one of the cæcal fossæ, an interesting observation on this subject was made by Scholt. He found the fossa closed at its mouth by adhesion similar in kind to those I have mentioned. The ultimate result of this closure was the formation of a cyst with clear contents.

The possibility of the analogous origin of a mesenteric cyst from the fossa of Waldeyer, to be presently described, should be borne in mind.

CHAPTER II.

THE DUODENAL FOLDS AND FOSSÆ.

IN describing the detailed anatomy of the various fossæ in this region, it is well to clear the ground a little by referring to the exuberant and redundant nomenclature that has been adopted by the various writers at different periods. The term that has perhaps been, on the whole, most subjected to abuse is 'duodeno-jejunal.' It has been applied indiscriminately to every variety of fossa found in this region, to fossæ which are strictly duodenal, to fossæ which are jejunal, and to fossæ which are neither. But more and worse than this is the adoption by one author of a name suggested by an earlier writer for a fossa quite different from that which is being described. The result is chaotic. In following out the descriptions applied by authors, one is being continually led away in thought by this process of name-appropriation. It must, however, be confessed that it is a matter of no little difficulty to find an exactly suitable name for each fossa, and it will be found that I have given, in almost every instance, an alternative title. In all cases the first title mentioned is in my opinion the aptest, and much perplexity would in future be avoided if that alone could be accepted.

HISTORY OF THE FOSSÆ.

The first mention, so far as I have been able to ascertain, of these fossæ is by Hensing (1742): 'In initio scilicet jejuni mesenterium versus renem sinistrum tendit, atque ascendo, finem mesocoli transversæ partis includit; antequam vero hoc præstat plicam quandam parvam, in qua concavitas latus sinistrum, convexitas vero latus dextrum respicit, constituit.'

It is no more than a brief allusion, and is, but for its antiquity, unimportant. Short reference was made to them also by, among others, Monro, who spoke of a 'ring,' Haller, and Sandifort.

The first description of importance, however, is that of Huschke (1844). He alludes to 'a triangular fossa at the junction of the duodenum and jejunum, which opens on the left side of the lumbar vertebræ, and is bounded above and

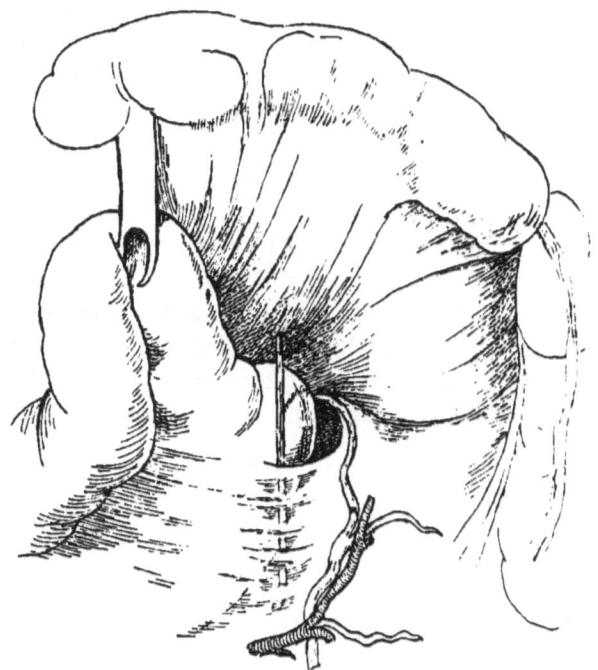

Fig. 3.—The Fossa described as Duodeno-Jejunal by Treitz.

below by two falciform processes of peritoneum which spring from the root of the transverse mesocolon.' Our knowledge is, however, chiefly derived from Treitz, whose great work was published in 1857. Before his time the subject of retro-peritoneal hernia practically did not exist. It was he who first recognised that such herniæ occur in fossæ which are normal, and it was he who first gave us any intelligent description of the fossæ and their probable mode of origin. He says: 'If in a body with a normal peritoneum one lifts up the great omentum and the transverse colon, and pushes over to the right the mass of small intestines, there will be seen on the left side of the duodeno-jejunal flexure a peritoneal fold (Fig. 3). This fold varies in shape and size. Most frequently it is semilunar, the thin concave edge looking upwards and to the right, and surrounding the bowel at the level of the flexure. The upper horn of this semilunar fold is blended with the inferior layer of the transverse mesocolon, and especially at the point where the inferior mesenteric vein passes beneath the pancreas. The larger lower horn is continuous on the inner side with the peritoneal investment of the duodenum, and at the outer

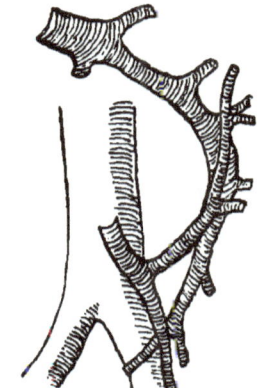

Fig. 4.—The 'Vascular Arch' of Treitz.

end with the peritoneum of the transverse and descending mesocolon. In the upper horn, at a variable distance from the edge, lies the inferior mesenteric vein, forming an arch, with the convexity looking upwards and to the left. The lower horn is less distinct, composed exclusively of two layers of peritoneum, and, at some distance from its free border, one sees the inferior mesenteric artery and its branch, the left colic artery. From the relative positions of these two vessels there results a vascular arch (always referred to now as the "Arch of Treitz") which surrounds the fold in question (Fig. 4). Behind this peritoneal fold—between it and the duodenum—there exists, necessarily, a depression or pocket in the form of a funnel, the summit of which is directed towards the duodenum. The orifice of entry is semilunar, limited on the right by the intestine, the flexura duodeno-jejunalis; on the left by the free border of the fold. This fossa is in general situated on the left side of the third lumbar vertebra.'

That is a brief epitome of his description. The next articles of importance were written by Wenzel Gruber, in 1859 and 1861. To the fossa described by Treitz he applies the cumbrous title 'retro eversio mesogastrica seu media, seu intermesocolica.' He mentions as variants a fossa showing three funnel-shaped divisions, and a division of the orifice of the fossa by fibrous bands. With regard to the arch of Treitz, he found it sometimes in front of the fossa in the anterior wall, sometimes behind, and sometimes distant on the outer side, a distance varying up to a maximum of 1 centimetre.

In 1862 Gruber published a record of three examples of a common mesentery for the small and large intestine. In one case, very beautifully illustrated, there existed a right inguinal hernia and an internal hernia, of the form which has lately been described as right duodenal. The existence of a right duodenal hernia he explained as being due to the right-sided position of the fossa duodeno-jejunalis of Treitz. The duodenum, instead of terminating on the left side of the spine, was in shape something like the letter S, and its junction with the jejunum lay to the right of the lumbar vertebræ.

In 1868 Waldeyer published an excellent description—the best up to that time—of the anatomy of the peritoneal fossæ. I shall attempt to show later how an important observation that he then made has been completely overlooked. The fossa duodeno-jejunalis of Treitz he found present in 73 per cent. of 250 cases consecutively examined. The size of the fossa varied considerably, being capable of containing sometimes only the terminal joint of the index finger, sometimes as much as 12 or 18 inches of small intestine.

The fossa was in some cases divided up by fibrous bands passing across the mouth. These bands were looked upon as abnormal, but, as shown by Toldt (see Chapter I.), they may be considered as additional 'fusion lines,' and not as the result of a fœtal peritonitis.

Eppinger, in 1870, published some important observations. It was said by Treitz and his followers that the vascular arch was always in close relationship with the folds bounding the opening into the fossa. Eppinger in 25 cases found the disposition to be as follows:

In 7 cases the vessels ran in the edge of the fold.

In 15 cases the vessels were distant 4 to 17 millimetres from the edge.

In 3 cases the vein lay behind the posterior wall of the fossa.

Eppinger applied the term 'incomplete' to fossæ which lacked the upper cornu (4 cases out of 11) or the lower cornu (7 out of 11). In these cases the arch of Treitz was distant 21 to 39 millimetres from the duodeno-jejunal angle. It will be shown later that in these cases Eppinger was referring to a fossa entirely separate and distinct from that of Treitz. Mention is also made, as by Waldeyer, of the subdivision of the fossa by fibrous 'adhesions' crossing the open mouth.

In 1871 Landzert added considerably to our knowledge by a most complete and interesting paper, which has never yet received adequate appreciation. He showed, first of all, that the relationship described by Treitz as existing between the vascular arch and the fold bounding the fossa is by no means necessary or even regular. As a rule, the vessels are placed some distance outside the margin of the fossa. In investigating the subject in the newly-born, Landzert showed that a large fossa was formed (separate from, as a rule, but capable of union with, the fossa of Treitz) on the posterior wall of the abdomen, by the raising up of a large fold by the inferior mesenteric vein and the left colic artery (Fig. 5). The fold, in fact, was practically a mesentery of these vessels. 'The fossa,' he says, 'is bounded above by a fold containing the inferior mesenteric vein, to the left by a fold containing the left colic artery, below by the mesenterico-mesocolic fold, and to the right by the mesentery of the small intestine.' The relations of this fossa with that of Treitz are well shown in a transverse section of the abdomen.

Wenzel Gruber, in one of his cases of duodenal hernia, had found that the mouth of the sac was bounded by these vessels in the manner described above. On removing all the intestine from the sac, he discovered, however, that behind and to the right of the mouth of the sac there was plainly to

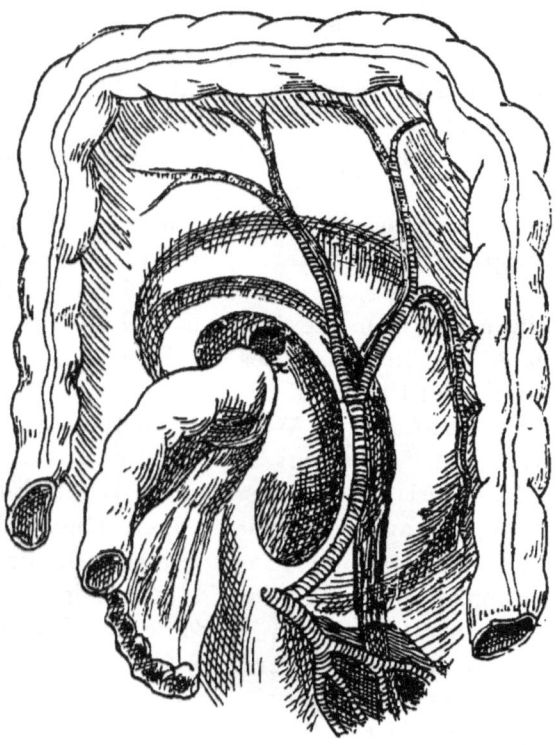

FIG. 5.—THE FOSSA OF LANDZERT AND THE FOSSA OF GRUBER (x). PARA-DUODENAL FOSSA AND POSTERIOR DUODENAL FOSSA.

be seen a second fossa (Fig. 5, x), a fossa which Gruber considered to be the fossa of Treitz. Landzert considered that his description of the anatomy of this region coincided with that given by Gruber; but it will presently be shown that both authors were construing the facts ill, that they were describing a fossa which until then had entirely escaped recognition. From Landzert's day up to 1890 the subject received little or no attention. In that year Jonnesco's work, to which I shall make frequent reference, was published.

He described therein three fossæ—a duodeno-jejunal, first described by Huschke, and a superior and inferior duodenal, corresponding to the upper and lower divisions of the fossa of Treitz.

It will be noticed that the number of the fossæ described had been increasing. From the one of Huschke and Treitz, the two of Gruber and Landzert, we come to the three of Jonnesco. In 1895 two other fossæ, a retro-duodenal and a para-duodenal, were mentioned by Jonnesco in Poirier's Anatomy. In 1891 there appeared a short work by Brösike of Berlin, dealing with the fossæ and the herniæ originating therein. This latter is the most thorough and complete work that I have met with. A full and generally accurate account is given of the anatomy of the fossæ and their folds. The letter-work is good, the illustrations are lamentably bad. Its terseness of style and compression of material contrast refreshingly with the redundancy and repetition of Jonnesco's work.

THE FOLDS AND FOSSÆ.

I propose to describe the following fossæ:

1. The superior duodenal fossa.
2. The inferior duodenal fossa.
3. The posterior duodenal fossa.
4. The duodenal-jejunal fossa.
5. The inter-mesocolic fossa.
6. The infra-duodenal fossa.
7. The para-duodenal fossa.
8. The mesenterico-parietal fossa, or fossa of Waldeyer.
9. The para-jejunal fossa of Brösike.

1. **The Superior Duodenal Fossa** (*Recessus duodeno-mesocolicus superior*, Brösike; upper horn of the fossa of Treitz—Fig. 6) is present in from 40 to 50 per cent. of cases. It may exist alone, or be present with the inferior duodenal fossa. It lies to the left of the ascending portion of the duodenum, near its termination. The orifice looks downwards, sometimes slightly to the right, sometimes slightly to the left,

opposing the mouth of the inferior duodenal fossa. The apex of the fossa extends upwards to the body of the pancreas. It is bounded in front by the *superior duodenal fold*, triangular in shape, presenting a lower free margin, slightly concave (semilunar), whose inner end is blended with the peritoneum on the anterior surface of the duodenum, and whose outer margin is lost on the mesocolon, near the

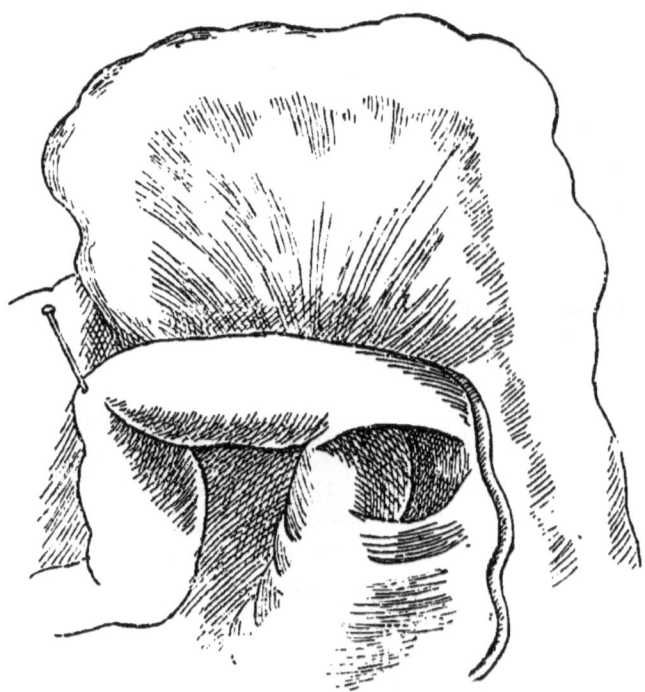

FIG. 6.—THE SUPERIOR AND INFERIOR DUODENAL FOLDS AND FOSSÆ.

junction of the transverse and descending, and in front of the left kidney. The upper part of the fold is continuous with the transverse mesocolon. To the right lies the duodenum, behind is the parietal peritoneum over the second lumbar vertebra, and the angle formed by the left renal vein and the aorta. The point of junction of the superior duodenal fold with the descending mesocolon may be within, correspond to, or be outside the inferior mesenteric vein; as a general rule, the vein corresponds almost exactly with this line of union. In fact, so frequent is this that Jonnesco describes the superior duodenal fold as 'always vascular.'

2. **The Inferior Duodenal Fossa** (*Fossa duodeno-jejunalis*, Treitz ; *Recessus duodeno-mesocolicus inferior*, Brösike ; *Fossa duodeno-mesocolica*, Toldt—Fig. 6).—This is the most frequent of all the peritoneal fossæ found in this region. It exists in from 70 to 75 per cent. of cases, being more or less well defined, sometimes quite distinct, sometimes a little difficult of recognition. In its typical form it may be thus described: it is situate on the left side of the ascending portion of the duodenum, opposite the third lumbar vertebra. The orifice looks almost directly upwards, with occasionally a slight lateral inclination ; it is opposed to the downward-looking mouth of the superior duodenal fossa. The fundus inclines downwards, practically always to the right, to the root of the mesentery. The fossa is bounded in front by the *inferior duodenal fold*. This fold in its characteristic form is triangular in shape. The upper margin is sharp and usually devoid of fat ; the inner end is lost on the anterior surface of the duodenum ; the outer end blends with the peritoneum covering the posterior abdominal wall. To the right of the fossa is the ascending portion of the duodenum, behind is the parietal peritoneum covering the third lumbar vertebra ; the apex of the fossa generally extends a little way down on to the fourth lumbar vertebra.

The inferior mesenteric vein and the left colic artery are generally found well to the left side of the point of fusion of the inferior duodenal fold with the descending mesocolon. In some cases, however, the vein, it is said, may be found in the free edge of the orifice ; and I have, though rarely, found the vein in the posterior wall of the fossa, internal to the outer margin of the fold. When the vein runs in the brink of the orifice of the fossa, it may have the left colic artery encircling it spirally.

Jonnesco then designates the fossa as the 'inferior duodenal vascular fossa,' or the 'fossa of Farabœuf' (Fig. 8). The more correct view, I believe, and one which I shall later explain, is to look upon these aberrations as due to an amalgamation of the inferior duodenal fold with the plica venosa, or mesentery of the inferior mesenteric vein. The inferior duodenal fossa then blends with the fossa of Landzert, the para-duodenal fossa of Jonnesco. The fossa varies very considerably in size and extent. Treves, in his Hunterian Lectures, described and figured several of the aberrant forms. In general the first joint of the middle finger can be conveniently passed within the fossa.

It is by no means infrequent to find the superior and inferior duodenal folds, when both are present, blending at their outer margins, so that the orifice bounded by the two is oval in shape. It results then in there being two fossæ with one mouth of entrance. Good examples of this kind are recorded by Waldeyer. Under such circumstances I have frequently observed that there is a very obvious extension of the fossa behind the ascending portion of the duodenum, so much so that the finger introduced into the fossa can be hooked round, so to speak, the left margin of the duodenum on to its posterior surface. This posterior extension of the cul-de-sac is seen occasionally when only the inferior duodenal fossa is present, but it is, in my experience, more frequent and of a greater extent in those cases where the upper and lower folds are blended. I have not been able to find anywhere a description of this extension of the fossa. This is very remarkable, seeing that in some cases it is strikingly obvious.

The junction of these folds may be looked upon as an excess of the normal process of physiological adhesion, and further evidence of this excess may be present in the form of one, or, as I have on a single occasion seen, two bands or peritoneal folds stretching across the mouth of the sac, thereby dividing the orifice up into two or three smaller openings.

3. **The Posterior Duodenal Fossa** (*Recessus duodeno-jejunalis posterior*, Brösike, or the fossa of Gruber—Fig. 5, *x*).—This is the fossa which I have briefly referred to as being seen by Gruber after the emptying of the sac of a left duodenal hernia, lying behind and to the right of the mouth of the sac. Gruber first described it as an 'accessory sac,' but later he considered it to be the fossa duodeno-jejunalis of Treitz, a mistake which was subsequently shared by Land-

zert. The fossa is carefully described by Brösike, who applies the name 'Recessus duodeno-jejunalis posterior' because 'in the normal position of the gut the fossa lies immediately behind the flexure.' It is, I believe, more strictly correct to say that the fossa lies immediately behind the upper portion of the ascending limb of the duodenum. The opening of the fossa is directed upwards and slightly to the left; its blind extremity is directed downwards and slightly to the right. It is bounded in front by the duodenum, and behind by the parietal peritoneum covering the lumbar vertebræ. On the right lies a fold of peritoneum, which contains, or rather covers, the 'musculus suspensorius' of Treitz. This fold is the *plica suspensoria*. To the left lies a fold, the *plica duodenalis posterior* or *plica duodeno-jejunalis posterior* (Brösike), which runs between the parietal peritoneum and the left side of the ascending portion of the duodenum. These two folds may vary from the perpendicular to the horizontal in direction. Landzert describes them as 'upper' and 'lower.'

The varieties of the fossa will depend no doubt, upon the greater or less degree of development or possible absence of either the one fold or the other. But one point is of vast importance. It is that the highest degree of completeness in this fossa is only found in association with the paraduodenal fossa. The cases of Gruber and Landzert are therefore the more readily understood.

The folds and the fossa result most probably from a fusion of the duodeno-jejunal flexure, and the adjacent portion of the duodenum, with the under layer of the transverse mesocolon. In the subsequent dragging of the duodenum slightly to the left, the folds are accentuated, and the fossa thereby deepened. The folds are therefore '*fusion folds.*'

4. **The Duodeno-Jejunal Fossa** (*Recessus duodeno-jejunalis superior oder die Jonnescosche Tasche*, Brösike; *Fossette duodénojéjunale ou mésocolique*, Jonnesco—Fig. 7).—This is the fossa which, as I believe, Huschke was the first to describe. In the article to which I have previously referred, he expressly states that the folds spring 'from the root of the transverse mesocolon,' a statement which is obviously untrue about all other folds.

On dragging the transverse colon upwards, and the jejunum downwards and to the right, there can be seen at the root of the transverse mesocolon a fossa, which results from the plunging, as it were, of the duodeno-jejunal flexure backwards into the root of the transverse mesocolon. This is the duodeno-jejunal fossa. It is found approximately in 15 to 20 per cent. of the bodies examined. Laterally, it is bounded by two folds—the duodeno-jejunal or duodeno-mesocolic folds (*plicæ duodeno-jejunalis superiores*, Brösike). These are, in reality, merely the continuations backward of the two leaves of the mesentery, which, skirting the duodeno-jejunal flexure, unite above it in a semilunar fold, whose edge looks

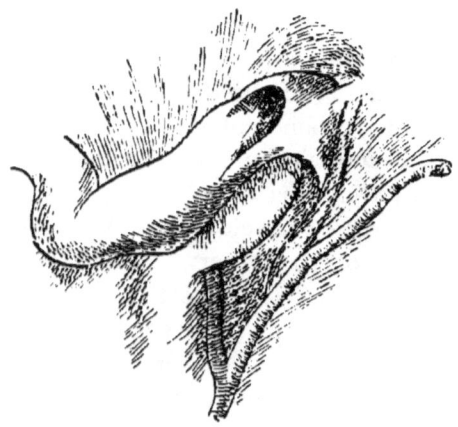

FIG. 7.—THE DUODENO-JEJUNAL FOSSA.

downwards and to the right. The fossa is bounded above by the pancreas, to the right by the aorta, to the left by the kidney. In the floor lies the left renal vein. The duodeno-jejunal flexure is a hernial content of the cul-de-sac. The inferior mesenteric vein running upwards and to the right forms a concavity, which corresponds with a fair degree of accuracy to the upper limit of the fossa. The fossa is always vascular.

In the cases where this fossa is found there has never yet been seen any other form of duodenal fossa.

In a few cases a division of the orifice of the sac by a peritoneal fold has been observed. This is probably produced in a similar manner to the division of the superior and inferior duodenal fossæ. Brösike, however, is inclined to believe that such division results from the raising up of a peritoneal fold by the inferior mesenteric vein, which crosses the mouth of the sac. I have never verified the description of a double-barrelled orifice, and therefore can offer no opinion on the point.

5. **The Inter-Mesocolic Fossa** (*Recessus inter-mesocolicus transversus*, Brösike; fossa of Brösike—Fig. 8).—This fossa,

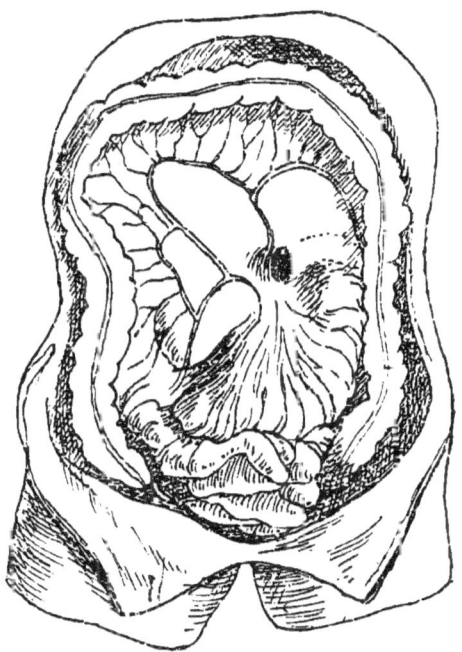

Fig. 8.—Recessus Inter-Mesocolicus Transversus. Inter-Mesocolic Fossa, or Fossa of Brösike.

first pointedly described by Brösike, is of rare occurrence. I have only once met with it, some years ago. I then made a rough sketch of it, but thought no more of the matter until I read the account given by Brösike. The fossa I observed corresponds quite accurately with those which he observed on the left side.

Brösike considers it as a modification of the fossa of Jonnesco just described. He has seen it six times—thrice on the left side, thrice on the right. It runs horizontally in the root of the transverse mesocolon. When placed as in the figure, the opening is downwards and to the right, and the blind extremity is to the left. The upper or hinder wall is formed by the transverse mesocolon and the pancreas; the lower wall by the upper portion of the ascending portion of the duodenum and the duodeno-jejunal flexure; the anterior wall by a special fold of peritoneum, uniting the under surface of the transverse mesocolon with the flexure and the line of attachment of the meso-jejunum. This fold Brösike terms the 'plica infra-mesocolica transversa.' The middle colic artery lies near the opening, to the right. In all his cases Brösike observed a marked deviation of the duodeno-jejunal flexure to the left, sometimes as far as the left kidney, and in the case figured almost to the descending colon.

The origin of the fossa is attributed to the formation of a fusion fold, the plica infra-mesocolica transversa, between the opposing surfaces of the transverse mesocolon on the one hand, and the duodeno-jejunal flexure and the meso-jejunum on the other.

This is the fossa which, no doubt, Toldt refers to when he mentions a right-sided duodeno-jejunal fossa, due to the fusion of the jejunum to the under layer of the transverse mesocolon.

6. **The Infra-Duodenal Fossa** (*Fossette retro-duodenale*, Jonnesco —Fig. 9).—This fossa, first described and figured by Jonnesco in 1893, is perhaps more conveniently, and equally accurately, described as 'infra-duodenal.' The term 'retro-duodenal' applies equally well to that offshoot from the combined superior and inferior duodenal fossæ which passes behind the ascending limb of the duodenum, and I am inclined to think that the term should be reserved for that offshoot. The orifice of this fossa looks downwards; its apex reaches the duodeno-jejunal angle, the muscle of Treitz, and the pancreas. It is bounded in front by the posterior aspects of the horizontal and ascending portions of the duodenum; behind, by the aorta, which projects into the cavity of the fossa, and laterally by two serous folds—the *duodeno-parietal folds*. These are triangular, having a base looking downward,

a duodenal border which is attached on each side to the posterior surface of the duodenum, and a parietal border which is blended with the posterior parietal peritoneum on each side of the aorta. At the line of fusion of the left ligament there lies the inferior mesenteric vein. The depth of the fossa varies from 7 to 9 centimetres.

7. **The Para-Duodenal Fossa** (*Recessus duodeno-jejunalis sinister, seu venosus*, Brösike; fossa of Landzert, Jonnesco—Fig. 10).—

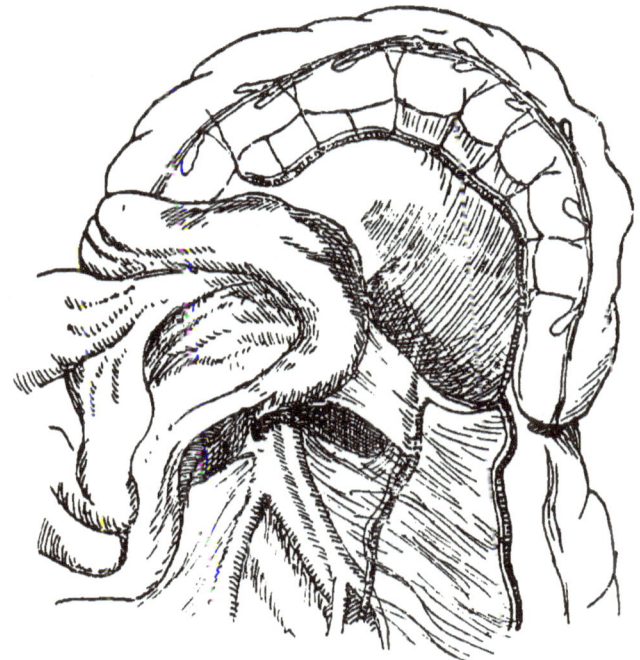

Fig. 9.—The Infra-Duodenal Fossa.

This is the fossa which was first accurately described by Landzert, though seen, without appreciation, by both Treitz and Gruber. In the first plate at the end of Treitz's work, the omission of the fold lying in front of the director would result in a quite characteristic fossa of this kind presenting. The point, however, which has caused the difficulty in understanding correctly the limits and boundaries of this fossa is that it exists not seldom in conjunction with other fossæ. The complications are almost as frequent as the normal. In its typical form, seen most frequently in the fœtus or the newly-born, the fossa may be thus described: It is situated to the left, and some distance from the ascending limb of the duodenum. The fossa is caused by the raising up of a fold, the plica venosa, by the inferior mesenteric vein—a fold which may be not inaptly described as a 'mesentery' of that vein. Behind, the sac is bounded by the parietal peritoneum, covering the psoas, the renal vessels, the ureter, and a portion

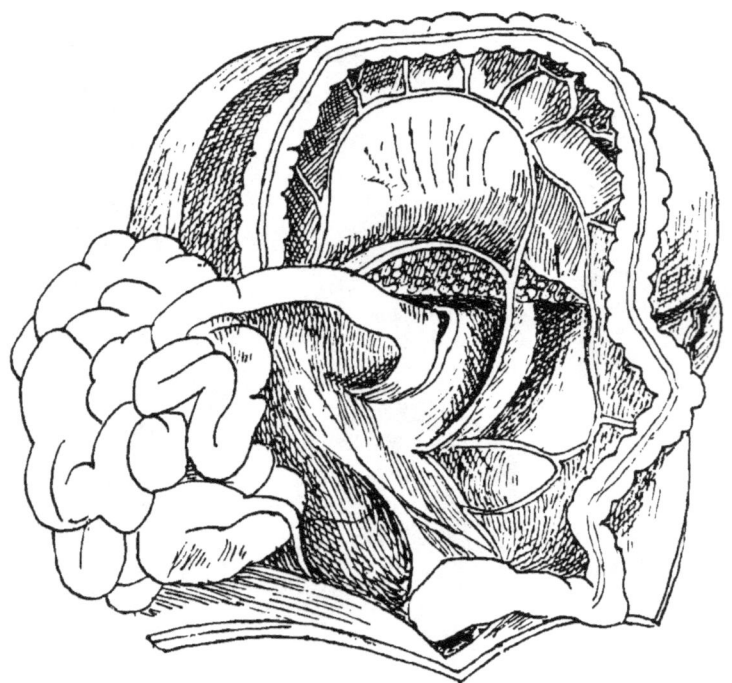

Fig. 10.—The Para-Duodenal Fossa.

of the left kidney. The orifice of the sac is wide, and looks downwards and to the right; the blind extremity is directed upwards and slightly to the left. The width of the orifice depends, of course, upon the distance between the inferior mesenteric vein and the duodeno-jejunal flexure, a distance which is capable of great variation. The plica venosa consists of a vertical and a horizontal portion, the vertical being to the left and below the fossa, and the horizontal bounding the fossa above. The inferior mesenteric vein forms a bow-shaped curve as it arches over to the right above the duodeno-jejunal flexure. Below, the fossa is limited by a serous fold the mesenterico-mesocolic fold, running from the left side of the mesentery downwards, and a little outward to the right side of the mesocolon of the upper portion of the omega loop.

In the case figured by Landzert (Fig. 5), there co-existed a small fossa at the duodeno-jejunal flexure (x) which he took to be the fossa of Treitz. It is more correct, as I have already said, to look upon this as the posterior duodenal fossa.

The inferior duodenal fossa may, however, be present at the same time as the para-duodenal fossa. When that is the case there is always an amalgamation of the two folds. A further deviation from the normal type of the fossa may be due to a firm agglutination of the horizontal limb of the plica venosa with the duodeno-jejunal flexure.

The description of this fossa that I have given differs in essentials from that of Jonnesco. Jonnesco describes the fold which I call the plica venosa as the mesentery not of the inferior mesenteric vein, but of the left colic artery. The outer margin of the fossa arches upwards and outwards, rather than downwards and inwards. In the case Jonnesco figures a second fold of peritoneum is raised transversely by the inferior mesenteric vein, dividing his para-duodenal fossa into an upper smaller and a lower larger segment (Fig. 15). I have never seen the form of fossa thus described, whereas the account I have given has been repeatedly verified.

For the origin and development of this fossa certain conditions are necessary.

As I have already stated, the fossa depends for its existence upon the formation of the plica venosa. In that early stage of development when the intestinal canal with its mesentery is mesially placed, the inferior mesenteric vein may occupy a variable position. It may be in the root line of the mesentery, or any distance away from this to the left towards the descending mesocolon. If not centrally placed, then, with the traction of the pancreas and the duodenum to the right, and the falling of the mesocolon away to the left, the vein will stand more or less prominently out, with a serous reduplication around it. I say 'more or less' because something depends upon the lax or taut condition of the vein between its origin and its point of union with the splenic or superior mesenteric vein. If a short course between these two points is run, then the vein is taut, and the peritoneal

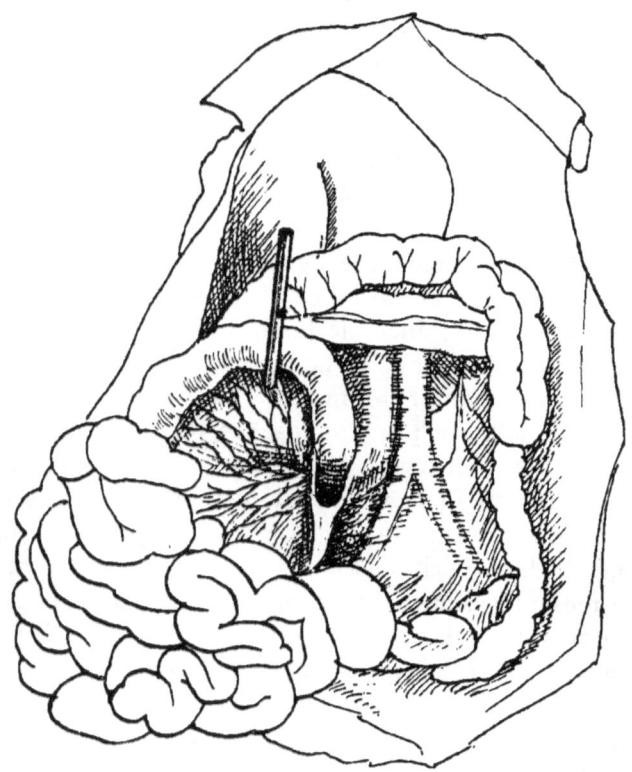

FIG. 11.—FOSSA PARA-JEJUNALIS OF BRÖSIKE, SHOWING JEJUNAL ADHESION.

fold raised by it the more prominent, and the fossa the deeper in consequence, and conversely. The fossa, then, and the fold which is responsible for it, are *vascular* in origin.

8 and 9. **The Mesenterico-parietal and the Para-jejunal Fossæ** (Figs. 11 and 12).—These may conveniently be studied together, for, in my opinion, they are practically the same fossa under different conditions.

The first mention of the mesenterico-parietal fossa, or fossa of Waldeyer, is contained in an article published by Waldeyer in 1874. The final paragraph of this paper has been consistently overlooked. It is to this effect: 'Finally, I will refer to the importance of the mesenteric vessels in the raising up of peritoneal folds and the formation of fossæ. Especially is this the case with the superior mesenteric artery, as it arches downwards with slightly concave curve to the right. I have not seldom, in embryos, found a fossa in the mesentery in the concavity of this arch. When the artery is prominent the fossa may be as much as half a centimetre deep, with its closed end directed downwards. I have found this fossa four or five times in fifteen embryos of fifteen to twenty weeks. At a later period it seems to be flattened

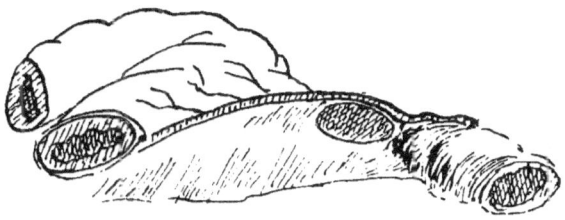

Fig. 12.—The Fossa of Waldeyer, lying behind the Superior Mesenteric Artery, and below the Duodenum.

out. In the adult I have never met such a condition; but it is noteworthy that already many cases of hernia into the mesentery and through "rents" in the same are described, for which, perhaps, this condition may afford an explanation.' In Sir A. Cooper's case of 'mesenteric hernia,' it was supposed that the sac was formed by the rupture of one layer of the mesentery and the entrance through the torn aperture of a segment of the gut, or else as the result of some defective development of the mesentery. Cooper says: 'If in consequence of a blow upon the abdomen one of these layers of peritoneum (of the mesentery) is torn and the other remains in its natural state, the intestines will force themselves into the aperture and form, according to my idea of the disease, a true hernia, since the intestine is protruded out of its proper cavity. Or, if either of these layers is originally formed defectively, so as to leave an aperture in one of them, the same effect will ensue. Which of these circumstances is the cause of the disease it is not in my power to determine; but I am disposed to believe that it has its source in an originally defective structure, as, in the case which I examined, there were no marks of preceding violence, but the parts had in all aspects, excepting in the existence of this disease, their natural appearance.'

The most usual position of this fossa is in the first part of the meso-jejunum, immediately behind the superior mesenteric artery, and immediately below the duodenum. The fossa varies considerably in size. I have not infrequently seen a slight, though well defined, bulging of the peritoneum in this situation, but I have only thrice met with a distinct fossa in adults. In seventeen embryos of less than five or six months I met with six fossæ. The fossa has its orifice looking to the left, its blind extremity to the right and downward. In front it is bounded by the superior mesenteric artery, and behind by the lumbar vertebræ. The peritoneum of the left leaf of the mesentery lines the fossa, that of the right covers the blind end, and is then continued directly into the posterior parietal peritoneum. A forcible enlargement of the fossa would thus result in a tearing up of this layer of peritoneum lining the posterior abdominal wall.

What I take to be the same fossa is differently described by Brösike, under the name 'recessus para-jejunalis.' He states that 'the recessus can only be present when the first portion of the jejunum is adherent for a longer or shorter distance to the posterior abdominal wall. I have seen this fossa only twice.' The first case is figured here (Fig. 11). ' In this the duodenum and the flexura duodeno-jejunalis were normal. From the flexure the jejunum ran obliquely downwards and to the right, adherent to the posterior abdominal wall, and devoid of mesentery. At the level of the fourth lumbar vertebra the mesentery began. On lifting up the first free portion of the jejunum, there could be seen behind and to the right of it a fossa, bounded by a sharp peritoneal fold, which, for want of a better term, I call the " plica para-jejunalis." On introducing the finger into the fossa, it could be felt to push its way between the mesentery and the posterior parietal peritoneum. There was no abnormality anywhere in the peritoneal cavity, but the free mesentery was strikingly long.' The second case occurred in a shrunken male subject, and was complicated by an abnormality in the position of the duodenum, but a similar fusion of the upper portion of the jejunum with the posterior abdominal wall was noted. On pushing a portion of gut into the sac, this latter increased in size by insinuating itself into the lax subperitoneal tissue.

Brösike attributes the origin of his fossa to an early fusion of the upper few inches of the jejunum with the anterior surface of the ascending limb of the duodenum, the result being that the upper portion of the common mesentery becomes slightly torn by the subsequent dragging in the movements of the intestine.

In support of Brösike's view of the causation of this fossa there may be quoted three cases of Treitz and two of Gruber's, and observations by His and Toldt. But that this posterior adhesion is by no means essential, or even usual, I shall subsequently attempt to show.

Such are the fossæ found in the duodenal region. Certain of them are found existing alone. The duodeno-jejunal, the infra-duodenal, and the fossa of Brösike are never found in conjunction with other of the fossæ. The fossa of Landzert, the para-jejunal fossa, on the contrary, is practically always found only when other fossæ are present, and, as I have said, its complications are almost as frequent as its normal condition. The most common union that it forms is with the inferior duodenal fossa, the fossa of Treitz. It was this blending which gave rise to the errors of description which have existed from the time of Treitz onwards.

I have described the fossæ in what I consider to be their normal and characteristic forms. It is important to remember that the fossæ and their folds are capable of considerable alteration. Not infrequently remnants of an old peritonitis are found, but all such cases I have left entirely out of consideration. Plastic adhesions so formed give rise to innumerable folds and fossæ. In all cases I have first made a general examination of the whole peritoneum, and only when no signs of old inflammatory mischief were present have I noted the condition of the fossæ. But in later life, apart from adhesive inflammation, certain changes are capable of being produced, by the continued dragging of parts, and especially by a large deposit of fat, which is in some cases so massive as entirely to obliterate all signs of folds or pouches. Of the influence of the intestinal traction on the shape of the fossæ, both Waldeyer and Toldt speak strongly. I have had unusually good opportunities of examining the fossæ in embryos and in children. In these, little alteration can have taken place, and I consider, therefore, that a description culled merely from observations in older subjects can hardly be considered typical. I shall make reference to this point in discussing one of the cases of hernia (Brösike's).

ORIGIN OF THE FOLDS AND FOSSÆ.

It is to Treitz that we are indebted for the first explanation that was given of the formation of the fossæ. He attributed their existence to the embryonic movement of the intestinal canal. 'It is the simultaneous displacement of the transverse mesocolon and the duodeno-jejunal angle which under certain circumstances causes the formation of the duodeno-jejunal fold and fossa.' The folds are attributed to the dragging of the intestine, in the displacement of the viscera to the right. They are, in fact, *traction folds*. The difficulty in accepting this theory lies in the fact, which Treitz himself was the first to demonstrate, that at a relatively early period—earlier, in fact, than the formation of the folds and fossæ—the duodenum is fixed by the suspensory muscle.

Waldeyer suggested the following explanation, based upon the idea of the close relationship of the fold and the inferior mesenteric vein. This vein is formed from the superior hæmorrhoidal and the left colic veins. At its origin it is closely applied to the posterior abdominal wall, but separates gradually from it as it ascends. It thus forms a sort of cord in the abdominal cavity. In proportion as the internal layer of the descending mesocolon disappears on account of the development of the left kidney, there is formed around the vein a sort of peritoneal fold, in the edge of which the vein runs. The fold then, according to Waldeyer, is *vascular*. This theory, plausible though it is, is based upon error, or, rather, upon a series of errors. The vein has not always, as Eppinger first showed, that relationship to the fold which Waldeyer considered essential, and, furthermore, the internal layer of the descending mesocolon, as I have previously said, is not disposed of in the manner described as normal by Waldeyer. With modifications to which I shall hereafter refer, this explanation is quite acceptable so far as the plica venosa alone is concerned.

The explanation given by Treves in his Hunterian Lectures is that the inferior duodenal fold represents the remains of the meso-duodenum, and is comparable to the duodenal fold of the hyena, which he figures. His theory entails a belief in the unfolding of the meso-duodenum. He says 'more peritoneum is required by the cæcum and ascending colon, and it is obtained from that of the posterior parietes, and in great measure by the unfolding of the meso-duodenum.' I believe, however, that the destiny of the meso-duodenum is that which I have described in the section on Development, and I therefore cannot accept as probable the hypothesis put forward by Treves. It is, moreover, not quite clear why, if these two structures, the meso-duodenum and the inferior duodenal fold, are identical, the free edge of the one should be at the upper limit, and of the other at the lower limit of the fold.

The interpretation of the genesis of the folds which I accept without hesitation is that they are to be looked upon as *fusion folds* between the original left, afterwards anterior, surface of the ascending portion of the duodenum and the right or anterior surface of the descending mesocolon folds, which date their origin from the time when these two peritoneal surfaces are in close opposition. Such a time is at the end of the third or the beginning of the fourth month. The line of fusion extends, in the case of the superior duodenal fold, from above downwards, and in the case of the inferior duodenal fold from below upwards. The line of agglutination becomes, by reason of the dragging of the duodenum in its journey to the right, and of the mesocolon in its tendency to the left, pulled upon and stretched, and at the expense most probably of the descending mesocolon the definite fold is formed. Toldt has stated that it is only in the eighth month of intra-uterine life that the folds are formed; but that they can not infrequently be found long before this I have repeatedly seen. Curiously enough, Toldt himself in one of his figures shows the folds quite distinctly developed in the fifth month. Indeed, I have verified on more than one occasion the following observation of Brösike's: 'In an embryo of the middle of the fourth month I found the two folds quite distinctly. As I drew the ascending portion of the duodenum gently to the right, I could see the two folds tear away quite easily from the anterior surface of the duodenum and disappear. There was here, quite obviously, a recent fusion present, which could not yet resist a gentle traction. In embryos of greater age the folds are capable of withstanding a far stronger pull.'

DUODENAL HERNIA.

Duodenal hernia is of two kinds. In the first and commonest the hernial sac increases to the left of the middle line, in the second to the right. In both cases there may be also an upward and downward increase, but the essential difference between the two forms lies in the varying direction of their lateral deviation. The left form of hernia is commonly described as 'duodenal hernia,' the differential term '*right* duodenal hernia' being employed to indicate that form which lies to the right of the middle line. This distinction should, I think, be accentuated by applying the terms 'right duodenal hernia' and 'left duodenal hernia' definitely to each variety, and this I propose to do. There is the greater justification for this, seeing that there is an intrinsic difference, not only in the mode of growth, but also, and chiefly, in the points of origin of the two forms. Moreover, the term at present in most common usage is 'duodeno-jejunal hernia,' which has nothing whatever to recommend it. For it is intended to convey the idea of the origin of the hernia in the inferior duodenal fossa a state of things which never occurs, and into the fossa which I have termed—following Jonnesco's example—'duodeno-jejunal' there is very possibly only one case of hernia on record, and that is not accepted as such by other authors. For every reason, then, the terms 'right duodenal' and 'left duodenal' are amply justified.

Left Duodenal Hernia.

Point of Origin.—The first point to be discussed is as to the particular fossa in which the hernial development takes place.

With regard to the superior duodenal fossa, it has been suggested by Jonnesco that this may be the sac of those cases of left duodenal hernia in which the enlargement takes place mainly between the layers of the transverse mesocolon. He suggests also that the duodeno-jejunal fossa may be the origin of similar cases. It is in the first place very unlikely that two fossæ, quite distinct in their position and formation, would give rise to one single variety of hernia. Furthermore, it would seem to be by no means an easy matter for intestine to enter either of these fossæ. The mouth of the superior duodenal sac looks directly downwards, and there would have, of necessity, to be a very great and probably a long-continued increase of intra-abdominal pressure to start the formation of a hernia. In the case of the fossa duodeno-jejunalis, I have already mentioned that in order to expose it satisfactorily a certain definite arrangement of the intestines is necessary. The transverse mesocolon must be tightly drawn upwards, and the jejunum downwards and to the right. It is only by doing this that the fossa can be made at all distinct. That either of these fossæ can commonly be the seat of a hernia is, then, very unlikely. There is, so far as I have seen, only one specimen of hernia that is in the least degree likely to have originated in the duodeno-jejunal fossa, and that is the 'mesocolic hernia' of Cooper.

After examining the original specimen in the St. Thomas's Museum, I am left in doubt as to the mode of origin; but of all other specimens that I have read of or examined there is no doubt possible upon one point. They cannot have had their origin in either of these fossæ.

The fossa of Brösike, the recessus inter-mesocolicus transversus, is never likely to develop any hernial contents. The fossa is exceedingly rare—Brösike has met with it on only six occasions, and I have met with it but once. Toldt has seen one case which may possibly have been a pouch of this description on the right side, and he suggested that in such a fossa a right duodenal hernia might find its origin. As I shall, however, point out later, a right duodenal hernia could not possibly have such an original position. When the fossa is well developed, it is only rather a potential pouch than an actual one. Its cavity can only be demonstrated by a careful dragging asunder of the meso-jejunum and the transverse mesocolon. Its orifice is directed downwards and the walls of it are in opposition. All these factors are quite against the possibility of the origin of a hernia here. But supposing such a hernia to occur, there would be an entirely different arrangement of vessels in the neck and anterior wall of the sac from any that I have yet met with.

With regard to the inferior duodenal fossa, or fossa of Treitz, it was for long supposed—and still the belief is universal—that all forms of duodenal hernia originate in this fossa. Treitz himself taught this, and later authors have implicitly accepted his views. Klob, who described a case of right duodenal hernia, expressed the opinion that such herniæ developed their sac at the expense of this pouch. Treves, in his Hunterian Lectures, says that all forms of duodenal hernia originate therein. Jonnesco gives a complicated description of the process by which a duodenal hernia originally left becomes eventually right. He believes that the fossa may be the sac, too, of a left hernia. The description of the vascular fossa of Farabœuf, given by him, shows clearly enough that there was here present a combination of the inferior duodenal and para-duodenal fossæ. Such a fossa he also considers as a potential sac of a left hernia. The typical inferior duodenal fossa, we have seen, is non-vascular, and the orifice of a hernial sac is always vascular. In the neck of such a sac can *always* be seen the inferior mesenteric vein. The left colic artery may be closely applied to it, or may be at some little distance away. (The two are very distinctly shown in a dissection of Pye-Smith's in the Guy's Hospital Museum.) But of the position of the inferior mesenteric vein in all the specimens I have examined there is no doubt whatever. It is true that in many of the cases that have been recorded the real essentials are mostly omitted, and especially is this the case with respect to any mention of the vein. In not a few of them the vein is not even named, yet I venture to say that it is of all points the one of chiefest importance. The fold containing the vein is the plica venosa, and the fossa bounded by such fold is the para-duodenal fossa, or fossa of Landzert. It is this fossa, then, that, so far as our present knowledge goes, forms the sac of a left duodenal hernia.

This para-duodenal fossa with its boundary fold, the plica venosa, was not seen or described in its own especial and particular form by Treitz, Waldeyer, or Eppinger. What Treitz described as the duodeno-jejunal fossa and fold were, I think there can be no doubt, the results of a confluence of the true inferior duodenal fold and fossa and the plica venosa and para-duodenal fossa. These two folds and their two fossæ exist quite independently of one another, are different in position, appearance, and modes of origin. But they not infrequently coalesce. Such coalescence results in a mixed form of fossa, which was observed and described by each of the great authorities I have named as an individual and peculiar form of fossa. That it is, however, merely the result of a coalescence of the two folds and fossæ the study of a very large number of cases has convinced me. I have had the good fortune to be able to examine the fossæ in more than thirty fœtuses, and in a fair number of children. It is in them that one meets with the clearest and most definite forms of fossa, for in them the conditions which I have earlier alluded to as giving rise to massive alterations of the fossæ have not yet occurred.

With regard, then, to the origin of a left duodenal hernia, it may be positively stated that the fossa which develops into the sac is in probably almost every case the para-duodenal fossa, or fossa of Landzert. The formation of a hernia in the superior duodenal fossa or in the duodeno-jejunal fossa is not denied. It is, however, exceedingly unlikely, and only one specimen that I have examined bears any evidence of such a mode of origin. That specimen is Sir Astley Cooper's 'mesocolic' hernia.

Conditions Predisposing to the Hernia.—The essentials which Treitz enumerated as being indispensable for the formation of a duodenal hernia are three, namely:

1. The existence of a fossa and its boundary fold.
2. The presence of the inferior mesenteric vein in the fold.
3. Freedom of movement in the small intestine to such an extent as to permit of its introduction into the hernial sac formed at the expense of the fossa.

In all the cases of left duodenal hernia that I have examined, or the reports of which I have carefully studied, three characteristics are invariably present. These are:

1. The presence of the inferior mesenteric vein in the neck of the sac. The extent of the margin actually formed by the vein varies somewhat in different specimens. In all, however, for a greater or less distance, generally greater rather than less, the vein is present and quite easily recognisable; for a portion of the distance it is usually placed in close relationship with the left colic artery.
2. The hernia spreads either outwards towards the descending mesocolon, or upwards into the transverse mesocolon, or both.
3. The hernial sac consists of a single layer of peritoneum. In its expansion away from the spine the sac will rest behind on the various structures placed on the posterior abdominal wall. In front of it will be the posterior parietal peritoneum, more or less closely united to the sac wall. It results then in the hernial contents having two layers of peritoneum in front of them and one layer of peritoneum behind them.

The Neck of the Sac.—The orifice of the sac is situated, as a general rule, at the back of the hernia, in close approximation to the lumbar vertebræ. Its exact relationship to the bulk of the hernia depends almost entirely upon the quantity of bowel contained therein. In the smaller herniæ it is situated to the right of the hernial mass, and looks slightly to the front. As the mass of bowel contained within the sac increases in quantity, the relative position of the orifice gradually becomes altered, becoming first right and eventually

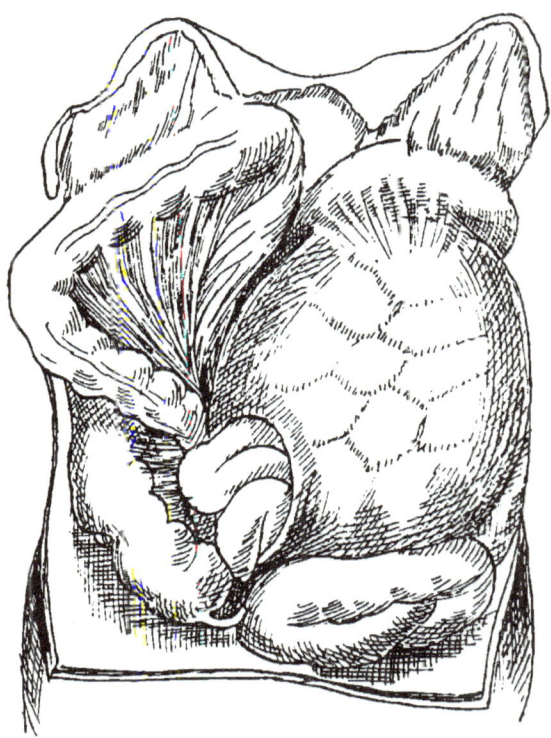

FIG. 13.—TREITZ'S CASE OF LEFT DUODENAL HERNIA.

right and posterior, and wholly posterior. In a large hernia it is necessary, in order to expose the neck of the sac, to drag the whole mass well over to the left side. The orifice is then seen close down to the third lumbar vertebra (Fig. 13). In the smaller herniæ the transverse measurement of the orifice generally exceeds the vertical, but with the increase in bulk the longitudinal diameter becomes more and more elongated, until eventually it may extend quite down into the neighbourhood of the cæcum. It is, however, not the largest herniæ which have always the largest orifices of entrance. Some very large herniæ have been seen where the neck of the sac was quite small, and *vice-versâ*. In many of the reported cases the size of the hernial orifice has been distinctly mentioned. Treitz records two where the aperture admitted in one case two, in the other three, fingers. Peacock's case admitted four fingers. Shattock's case would admit two with difficulty.

The following table, drawn up by Jonnesco, gives the accurate measurements as recorded by the observers of each case:

Length.	Breadth.	Observer.
$1\frac{1}{2}$ to 2 centimetres.	—	Lambl.
4 ,,	—	Krauss. Lambl.
$4\frac{1}{2}$ to 5 ,,	$3\frac{1}{2}$ centimetres.	Lambl.
6 ,,	3 ,,	Landzert.
6 ,,	3 ,,	Eppinger.
6 ,,	5 ,,	Eppinger.
7 ,,	5 ,,	Treitz.
7 ,,	6 ,,	Eppinger.
9 ,,	$7\frac{1}{2}$,,	Landzert.
13 ,,	$6\frac{1}{2}$,,	Gruber.

The opening of average size would be 6 centimetres long and 4 centimetres broad.

The orifice of the sac is bounded behind by the peritoneum of the posterior abdominal wall. Its boundary wall is here flat, and very frequently a pad of adipose tissue, more often well-defined, is found beneath the peritoneum.

The upper, anterior, and lower boundaries of the opening are formed by the edge of the peritoneal fold containing the inferior mesenteric vein, the plica venosa. At the lower part of the neck this border is generally thickened by a fatty deposit, but anteriorly and above the edge is sharp and thin. The left colic artery is generally closely applied to the inferior mesenteric vein throughout the whole of the anterior portion of the fold, but above the artery inclines upwards and a little to the left, while the vein arches boldly to the right. At the mouth of the sac there is always seen that portion of the intestine which is leaving the sac to be continuous with the small intestine, if any, between the sac and the cæcum. In the first case of duodenal hernia recorded, that of Neubauer, this arrangement was found (Fig. 14). No entering coil of intestine is seen, only the retiring segment. In other cases both entering and retiring coils are seen;

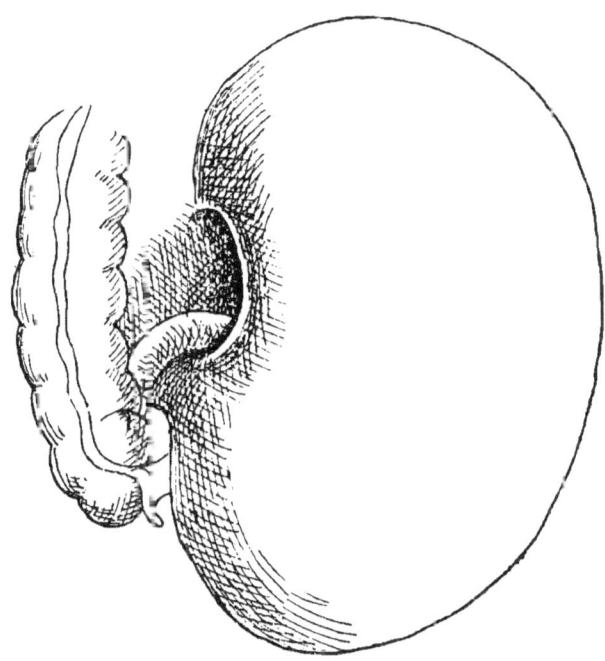

Fig. 14.—Neubauer's Case of Left Duodenal Hernia.
This is the first recorded.

and in some cases, though rarely, it has been found that coils enter and leave, re-enter and re-leave the sac.

The explanation of the condition met with by Neubauer, and in several later cases, must be this: The inferior mesenteric vein arches *over* the duodeno-jejunal flexure to its termination. Then, as the result probably of a process of 'physiological adhesion,' but possibly by a similar process which is pathological, there occurs a fusion—an agglutination of the mouth of the hernial sac with the anterior wall of the duodenum and of the duodeno-jejunal flexure. The result is that the highest portion of intestine contained within the sac, the duodeno-jejunal flexure, seems to come, not through the mouth of the hernia, but through the actual wall of the sac, on the right and posterior aspect of which it lies. The only tube of intestine, then, seen leaving by the orifice of the fossa is the lower end, that nearest the cæcum. In Neubauer's case practically the whole small intestine lay in the sac, for the bowel leaving the hernia was only an inch or two above the cæcum.

The Size of the Hernia.—The size of the hernia varies enormously. In some cases it is no larger than a walnut, in others practically the whole abdomen is filled. The length of intestine engaged in the hernia varies from 5 centimetres (Treitz), 4 or 5 inches (Shattock), up to the total length of the free small intestine. Several of the smaller specimens were observed by Treitz, Gruber, and Lambl, in autopsies performed upon children. In one case of Brösike's, occurring in a child fourteen days old (the youngest case on record), only 2 to 3 centimetres lay in the hernial sac. The fossa, however, was capable of holding about 8 centimetres. (In this case the plica venosa and the inferior duodenal fold were both present, and very clearly developed. This bears out what I have already remarked as to the distinctness of these fossæ and their folds in the earlier years of life.) As a rule, with very few exceptions, it may be stated that the older the subject, the larger the sac. The majority of the cases recorded are cases of complete, or almost complete, herniæ (where the whole or the larger portion of the small intestine lay in the sac), and they occurred in people at or well beyond adult age.

Jonnesco gives the following table, showing the size of the hernia in some of the smallest cases recorded :

Vertical measurement.	Transverse measurement.	Reporter.
$2\frac{1}{2}$ centimetres.	$1\frac{1}{2}$ centimetres.	Gruber.
8 to 10 ,,	—	Lambl.
11 ,,	14 ,,	Gruber.
14 ,,	12 ,,	Lambl.
18 ,,	12 ,,	Krauss.
20 ,,	$16\frac{1}{2}$,,	Krauss.
$24\frac{1}{2}$,,	$14\frac{1}{2}$,,	Gruber.

Jonnesco divides the herniæ into three classes according to their size—the small, the medium-sized, and the large. As there is no apparent reason for this purely arbitrary division, I see no advantage in adopting it.

The hernia, when small, has the following relations: It rests upon the psoas muscle, the inner portion of the kidney, the renal vessels, and above may reach to the pancreas.

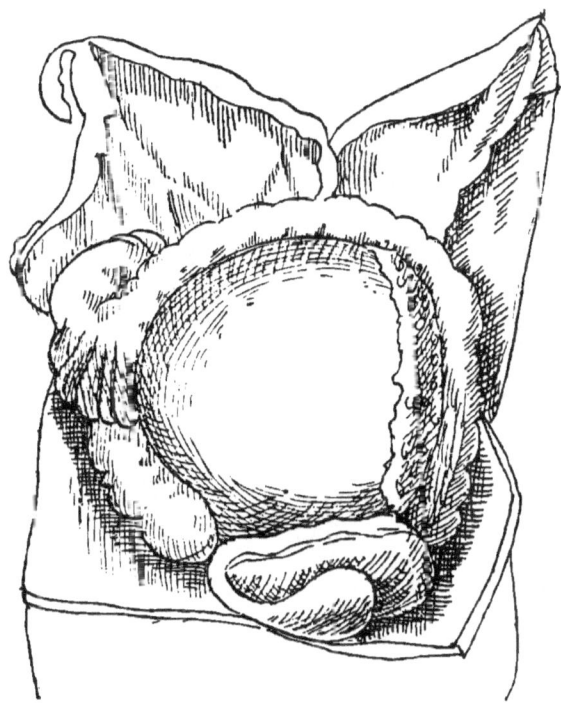

FIG. 15.—LEFT DUODENAL HERNIA, SHOWING THE COLON SURROUNDING THE SAC. (TREITZ.)

Internally lie the lumbar vertebræ and the aorta, and below the hernia reaches approximately to the lower end of the kidney. As the hernia increases in size, it enlarges outwards, or outwards and upwards, and comes to lie over the tail of the pancreas and the spleen. On the left side it reaches the descending colon, and below descends to the level of the bifurcation of the aorta.

In a further increase, the position assumed by the hernia

depends upon the anatomical condition of the descending mesocolon. If the process of physiological agglutination to which I have previously referred has been carried to its fullest extent, there is no mesocolon. In that case a hernia bulging outwards will push the colon at first outside, and finally (though rarely) behind it. The transverse and descending

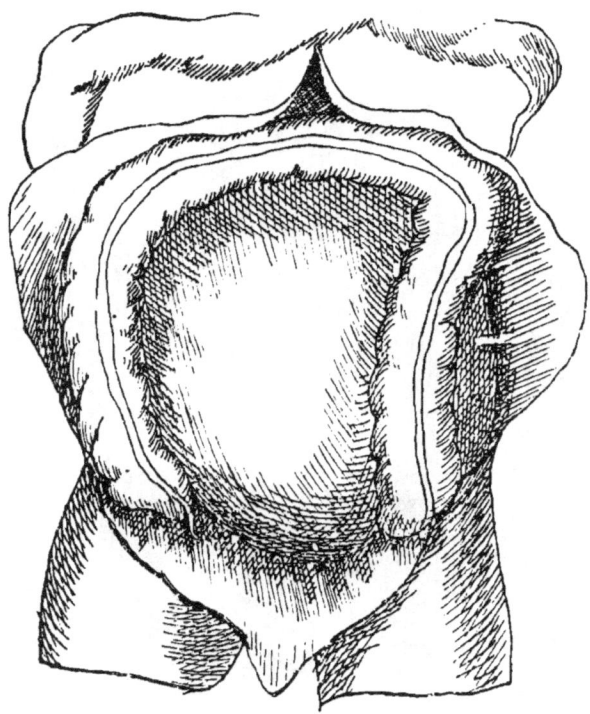

Fig. 16.—Left Duodenal Hernia, pushing the Outer Side of the Descending Colon. (Neubauer.)

colon then retain approximately their normal relative positions. The hernia is situated in the middle of the abdominal cavity, and the colon surrounds the mass (Fig. 15). If, however, the process of physiological agglutination has been less complete, a more or less perfect mesocolon will remain. In this case the mesocolon will be 'used up' by the oncoming hernia, and its layers will be spread out on the anterior wall of the sac. The hernial mass then gets outside and beyond the line of the descending colon, and in its subsequent enlargement pushes this downwards and to the right (Fig. 16). The transverse and descending colon may then be found either at the left, or, in extreme cases, at the lower and right portion of the anterior sac wall. The splenic flexure of the colon is then approximated to the cæcum (Fig. 17), or the colon may be found at any point between the two. Under

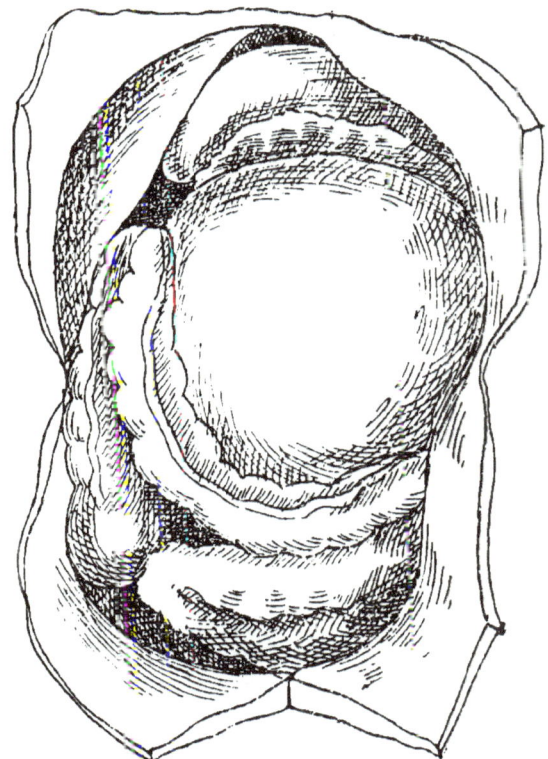

Fig 17.—Left Duodenal Hernia.

The sac has pushed its way above and to the outer side of the splenic flexure, which lies near the cæcum.

all circumstances, however, the cæcum and ascending colon are in great measure unaffected. They may be pushed a little away from the centre of the abdomen towards the periphery; but their relative positions remain unchanged, and the peritoneum in connection with them is undisturbed.

In its gradual augmentation in size, the hernia will be

affected by (1) the degree of laxity of the retro-peritoneal tissue ; (2) the extensibility of the peritoneum.

1. The sub-peritoneal tissue is the stratum in which the hernial sac rests, and from the first the increase in size of a hernia is due to the sac pushing its way in and among this generally lax membrane. If for any reason the sub-peritoneal tissue should be unusually dense, fibrous, inelastic, or inexpansible, to so much greater a degree will the increase of the hernia be impeded. The more loose and lax the tissue, the more rapid and the easier will be the accession of bulk.

2. So far as concerns the extensibility of the peritoneum, there is little to be said. In the absence of any adhesions the result of old peritonitis, the membrane lends itself readily enough to any increase of size of an intra-abdominal tumour, wherever originating.

History.—The cases recorded in surgical literature that I have been able to gather together number fifty-seven.

The authors are:

Neubauer (1776)	... 1 case.	Gruber (1862)	... 9 cases.
Bordenave (1779)	... 1 ,,	Breisky (1862)	... 1 case.
A. Monro, jun. (1803)	... 1 ,,	Waldeyer (1868)	... 1 ,,
Astley Cooper (1807)	... 1 ,,	Chiene (1868)	... 1 ,,
Cruveilhier (1827)	... 1 ,,	Gontier (1869)	... 1 ,,
Hesselbach (1829)	... 1 ,,	Eppinger (1870)	... 3 cases.
Hauff (1832)	... 1 ,,	Landzert (1871)	... 2 ,,
Soverini (1846)	... 1 ,,	Pye-Smith (1871)	... 1 case.
Peacock (1849)	... 2 cases.	Anderson (1872)	... 1 ,,
Barth (1849)	... 1 case.	E. Muller (1881)	... 1 ,,
Deville (1849 and 1851)	... 2 cases.	F. Krauss (1884)	... 2 cases.
Ridge and Hilton (1854)	... 1 case.	Shattock (1885)	... 1 case.
Treitz (1857)	... 8 cases.	Staudenmayer (1886)	... 1 ,,
Brugnoli (seen in 1846, reported 1859)	... 1 case.	Strazewski (1888)	... 1 ,,
		Brösike (1891)	... 1 ,,
Lambl (1860)	... 6 cases.	Tubby (1898)	... 1 ,,

A second case of Sir A. Cooper's, that described by him as a 'mesenteric' hernia, is also generally included. I am becoming increasingly confident in my belief that this is an example of the right duodenal variety.

A fuller reference is given at the end, in the Alphabetical List of References.

I have recently received the account of an unpublished case observed by Dr. Louis Mitchell of Chicago. Through his courtesy I am enabled to report it here.

'Mrs. M. T., aged thirty, coloured, was shot through the heart, dying immediately. At the necropsy, on making the usual median incision and cutting through the abdominal walls, instead of coming upon the omentum or the intestines, a white glistening sac was found which seemed at first to be a mesenteric cyst or an ovarian tumour. After reflecting the abdominal walls and tracing the relations, however, it was discovered to be a case of retro-peritoneal hernia.

'The mass, which measured 17·5 by 27 centimetres, reminded one of the gravid uterus, except that it was flattened in front. It was situated in the centre and left side of the abdomen, surrounded by the colon, extending below nearly to the promontory of the sacrum. The omentum, which was very thin and but slightly developed, was rolled up between the sac and the transverse colon. At the lowest aspect of the sac on the right was an elliptical opening 5 by 7·5 centimetres, from which 10 centimetres of the lower part of the ileum escaped obliquely to join the cæcum. The remainder of the small intestine was contained within the sac.

'The sac was smooth and shining, the walls thick but translucent, so the intestinal coils could be discerned; the walls of the sac contained numerous bloodvessels, but little fat. The sac was free except on the left and above, and several folds ran off from its border and were lost in the surrounding peritoneum.

'The orifice of the sac was situated low down close to the cæcum, and looked forward and to the right. The upper margin of this orifice was thick, fibrous, and opaque, becoming thinner below. The inferior mesenteric vein bordered the opening; the colica sinistra artery ran at some little distance from the free border; the vein was about the size of a goosequill.

'The coils of intestine in the sac were patent and moderately distended with gas, but were strongly adherent, so only part of them could be pulled out. The part that was motile showed no changes in the mesentery, or in the bowel itself.

'As regards the large intestine, the cæcum, ascending and transverse colons were in their proper places; the descending colon was in front of the sac, having been pushed forward; the rectum was normally situated. There was no congestion of the abdominal viscera or hæmorrhoid.

'Nothing abnormal was noted in the outward appearance of the abdomen. The walls were somewhat pendulous, but, as striæ were visible, this may have been due to past pregnancies. . . .

'Opinions differ as to the frequency of occurrence of the fossa. Thus, Waldeyer gives 70 per cent., Gruber 66 per cent., Treves 48 per cent., Debierre 50-75 per cent., and Jonnesco 75 per cent. for the inferior and 50 for the superior. I have examined 1,000 fresh adult bodies with a view to ascertaining in how many it was present, with the following results:

Males.		Females.	
Bodies examined	... 821	Bodies examined	... 179
Absent	... 513	Absent	... 101
Total	... 308	Total	... 78

'The results were less than those quoted, but the fossa was carefully searched for, and nothing counted as such unless it admitted the finger-tip.'

Right Duodenal Hernia.

Point of Origin.—A right duodenal hernia (*hernia mesenterico-parietalis*, Brösike) occupies in its earlier stages the right half of the abdominal cavity. When a large size has been attained, the sac may push its way over to the left side, and finally occupy equally the two halves of the body. A distinction has always been drawn between the two forms of duodenal hernia, left and right. The complete difference between their appearances during the earlier stages of development would account for this. Up to the present, however, I believe that no correct explanation, no lawful interpretation of the facts often observed, has been suggested.

The first hernia which is certainly of this variety was discovered and recorded by Klob on June 12, 1861, in the body of a male aged thirty-six years. (Sir A. Cooper's mesenteric hernia is assumed to be open to doubt.) The hernia is thus described: 'On opening the abdomen, one could see nothing of the small intestine. After turning up the great omentum and the transverse colon, there appeared, occupying the right half of the abdominal cavity, reaching to the middle line, a sac 8 inches long, 6 inches wide, and 5 inches deep. The upper portion was covered by the transverse mesocolon. To the right lay the ascending colon. Below, the sac lay in the pelvis. The orifice of the sac lay to the left and behind, was about 2 inches in diameter, and was situated on the third lumbar vertebra. In the thin anterior margin of the orifice lay the ileo-colic artery.' The explanation of the origin of this hernia given by Klob is that the sac developed at the expense of the inferior duodenal fossa of Treitz. This view has been adopted by Jonnesco in his work in the following words: 'I believe the hernia (right duodenal) to be produced in the inferior duodenal fossa, the non-vascular form, in which the summit touches the root of the mesentery. The ascending portion of the duodenum lies against the anterior or external wall of the fossa. The duodeno-jejunal angle, ill-supported by the muscle of Treitz, droops, and thereby predisposes to a prolapse of the ascending portion of the duodenum. This descends, pushing before it the inferior duodenal fold. Little by little the serous sac becomes pushed from left to right, and from above downwards. The fossa not having any immediate relationship to the vascular arch of Treitz, the serous sac, in place of ensconcing itself under the arch, misses it altogether. The increase of the hernia occurs in the direction of least resistance. I have frequently found an abundance of loose cellular tissue at the root of the mesentery. The apex of the fossa will therefore find no difficulty in pushing its way into the root of the mesentery, and it is then directed to the right.' This is pure hypothesis, with no single observation to support it. Indeed, it is directly contrary to fact, for in more than one carefully recorded instance the inferior duodenal fold has been distinctly noted to be present in cases of this form of hernia (Neumann).

Gruber, in recording his cases of common mesentery for the whole of the small and large intestine, explains the origin of a right duodenal hernia as being due to an anomaly in the position of the duodenal fossa. An arrangement, however, based upon such a grossly unconventional series of cases can have absolutely no weight when applied to cases with a normally attached mesentery. Moreover, there is no recognised variation in the situation of either the superior or inferior duodenal pouches.

Landzert attributed the origin to a fossa found by him in addition to his para-duodenal fossa. This new sac he considered to be the fossa of Treitz, but as I have already shown, the pouch he was describing was that which I have dealt with under the name of posterior duodenal fossa. This theory of origin need not be considered. The vascular relations of all right duodenal herniæ negative it absolutely and unconditionally.

Brösike has insisted that the one essential for their development is a fusion of the upper few inches of the jejunum to the posterior abdominal wall. This fusion is due to an excess of the process of physiological agglutination that I have referred to earlier in this work. As a result of the fusion a rent occurs in the mesentery, which later develops into a fossa situated in the uppermost portion of the meso-jejunum. In all cases that Brösike investigated he alleges that this abnormality was, and must be, present. Without it there could be no hernia. I shall presently show that this view is not universally applicable.

Toldt suggested that a fossa which on one occasion he saw at the right of the transverse mesocolon, near its junction with the ascending mesocolon, might be a dislocated pouch of Treitz. I have elsewhere remarked that what he saw was very probably that very rare fossa, the fossa of Brösike, the recessus inter-mesocolicus transversus.

Conditions Predisposing to the Hernia.—The factors which are, so far as I have been able to ascertain, invariably present in cases of right duodenal hernia are:

CONDITIONS PREDISPOSING

1. The hernial sac occupies—at any rate, at first—the right half of the abdominal cavity, lying behind the ascending and transverse mesocolon.

2. The orifice is situated behind and to the left of the sac, on the lumbar vertebræ.

3. In the anterior margin of the sac there lies either the superior mesenteric artery or a continuation of it, the ileocolic artery.

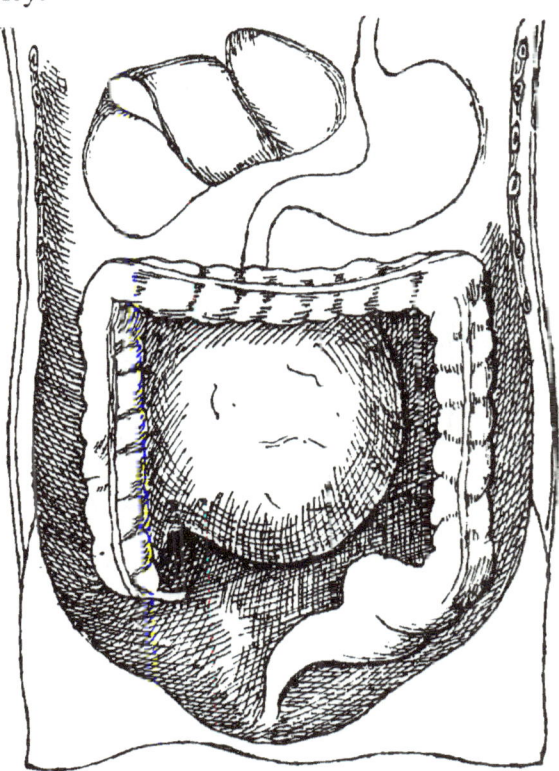

FIG. 18.—RIGHT DUODENAL HERNIA.
The sac is surrounded by the colon.

The Neck of the Sac, etc.—Now, I have already shown that in exactly the situation where the hernial sac first begins its development there is not infrequently in embryos, and occasionally in adult life, a fossa situated in the mesentery of the upper part of the meso-jejunum. This fossa was first described by Waldeyer, but his description has since been persistently overlooked. I propose to call the pouch the 'fossa of Waldeyer.' This fossa lies within the concavity of the arch formed by the superior mesenteric artery; its orifice looks to the left, its fundus to the right and downwards. Behind it are the lumbar vertebræ covered by peritoneum. Any intestine entering this pouch would develop a hernia fulfilling all the requirements of a right duodenal hernia. As it enlarges

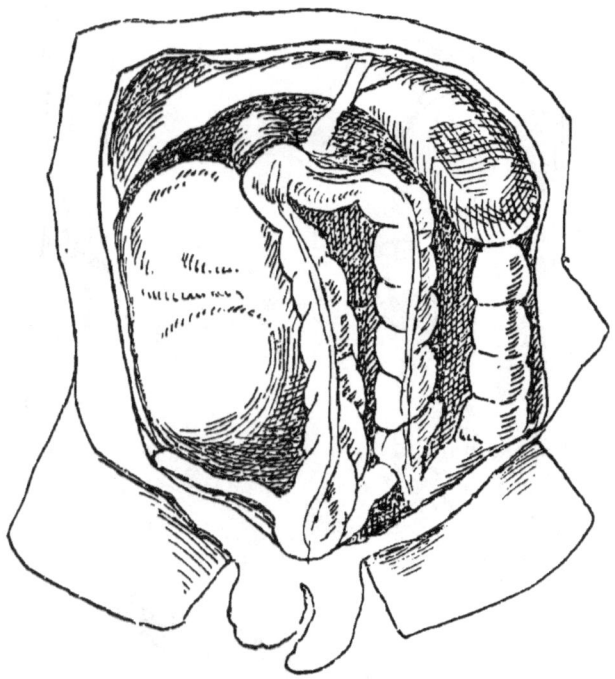

FIG. 19.—RIGHT DUODENAL HERNIA. (BRÖSIKE.)
Sac on the outer side of the ascending colon.

towards the right and upwards or downwards, this form of hernia would behave in a manner precisely identical with the left variety. The posterior parietal peritoneum would be stripped up until the colon was reached. Then either the colon would be pushed away from the tumour until the latter lay surrounded by the arch of the colon, as in Clarke's case and in Gerard-Marchant's case (Fig. 18), or if an ascending mesocolon were found this would be spread out over the anterior surface of the sac, and the hernia, passing behind the colon, would appear on its outer side, as in Brösike's case (Fig. 19).

It so happens that I have had the opportunity of closely examining two cases of this kind. The first was a case of the late Mr. McGills, in which Dr. Barrs performed the post-mortem examination, and subsequently reported in the *Lancet* of 1891. The following account is given : ' On opening the body in the ordinary way, one at once came upon what appeared to be a second sac of peritoneum containing apparently the whole of the small intestines, which could be seen distinctly through its walls. This sac was quite as large as an adult head (Fig. 26). It appeared to be free towards its upper left and lower limits, so that one's hand could be passed around it in these directions, but attached in all its parts to the right. It could be easily displaced or turned over to the right side, when a large aperture leading to its interior was at once exposed, and coils of distended small intestine began to escape. The hepatic flexure of the colon with the immediately adjacent parts of the ascending and transverse colon were incorporated in the right and upper part of the sac. The whole of the small intestine from the end of the duodenum to the ileo-cæcal valve was contained in the sac. In the anterior margin of the sac ran the superior mesenteric artery.' The jejunum was not adherent to the posterior abdominal wall. The facts were wrongly interpreted, but the vivid accuracy of the description leaves no doubt whatever that the case was one of right duodenal hernia. Dr. Barrs sent an account of the case to Mr. Treves, who identified the hernia as being allied to Sir A. Cooper's case of 'mesenteric hernia.' The duodeno-jejunal fossa was stated to be the sac of origin of the hernia. This case, which I carefully examined at the time, entirely negatives the statement of Brösike as to the inevitableness of the jejunal adhesion to the vertebræ. In the figure showing the orifice of the sac (Fig. 20) can be seen the transverse portion of the duodenum, tied and cut across. This portion of the duodenum then was fixed in the posterior and upper part of the neck. The fossa of Waldeyer lies normally below the duodenum, but evidently here the fossa has been enlarged by the rolling away of the peritoneum up to the superior mesenteric artery in the process of 'wandering' of the hernial orifice. This artery, emerging from beneath the pancreas, crosses the duodenum, and in the increase of the fossa in this direction the duodenum becomes more and more uncovered, until the whole of the anterior wall of the orifice of the sac is bounded immediately by the artery quite up to the point of its emergence. The duodenum then, from forming the upper boundary of the fossa, comes to lie in its posterior wall at the upper extremity. This explanation of

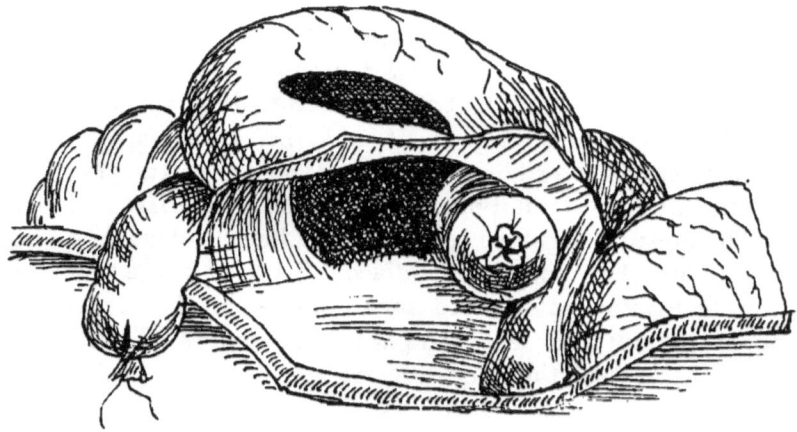

FIG. 20.—RIGHT DUODENAL HERNIA. (BARRS.)
Orifice of the sac formed by the fossa of Waldeyer.

the enlargement upwards of the orifice is more than plausible, for a precisely similar occurrence is noted so far as the lower boundary of the aperture is concerned. Every intermediate stage between the condition where the aperture has the appearance presented by Dr. Barrs' case to that presented by the case of Gerard-Marchant (Fig. 21) has been observed. In this case, the most extreme of its kind, the whole of the mesentery of the small intestine sprang from the anterior margin of the orifice of the sac. This enlargement of the neck of the sac until the orifice reaches the cæcum is in every respect comparable with and parallel to the extension upwards and unrolling of the peritoneum that I have described. The neck of the sac, in a word, behaves in a precisely similar fashion to the neck of every other hernia sac. The orifice enlarges almost or quite in proportion as the sac enlarges. Cases very similar to this one have been reported by Jackson Clarke and Neumann. Neumann's case has the additional interest attached to it that operation

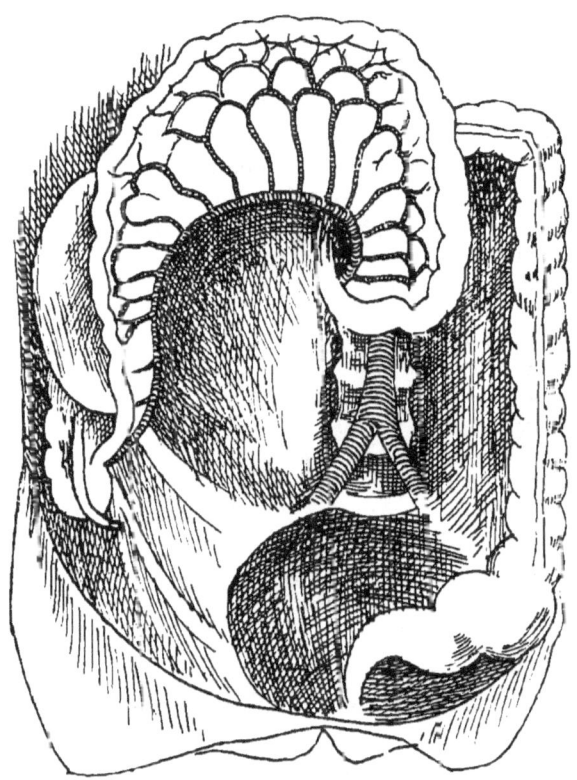

FIG. 21.—RIGHT DUODENAL HERNIA, SHOWING THE ORIFICE OF THE SAC BOUNDED BY THE SUPERIOR MESENTERIC AND ILEO-COLIC ARTERIES. (GERARD-MARCHANT.)

during an attack of acute obstruction was followed by recovery. So far this is the only case of recovery on record.

The second case, which I have examined closely, is one which has been preserved for some years in the post-mortem room of the Leeds Infirmary by Dr. Griffith. The history of the patient is not recorded.

The case is a most typical one. The hernial sac passes behind the superior mesenteric artery, and gets to the outer side of the ascending colon, which has a distinct, well-defined mesentery about 1 inch in length. The whole of the small intestine, from the duodenum to the cæcum, is contained in the sac. There is no jejunal adhesion to the posterior abdominal wall. The orifice of the sac is bounded by the superior mesenteric artery and its continuation, the ileo-colic, and extends from the duodenum to the ileo-colic angle. There is no trace of any pathological process in the sac. The intestines enter and leave quite freely.

Enumeration of Cases.—I have been able to get together the following authentic cases of right duodenal hernia:

Klob (1861)	1 case.
Gruber (1862)	1 "
Gerard-Marchant (Jonnesco)	1 "
Quenu (Jonnesco)	1 "
Furst (1884)	1 "
Zwaardemaker (1884)	1 "
Moutard Martin (1874)	1 "
Brösike (1891)	2 cases.
Jackson Clarke (1892)	1 case.
Barrs (1891)	1 "
Griffith (1898)	1 "
Neumann (1898)	1 "
Guy's Museum (No. 1084)	1 "
Total	14 cases.

I am also very strongly inclined to think that Sir A. Cooper's case of 'mesenteric' hernia is of the right duodenal variety, but as no accurate description of the orifice of the sac, its position, and boundary vessels is given, I have deemed it prudent to omit it. The case in Guy's Hospital Museum is called 'subcæcal.' Dr. Pye-Smith refers to it at the end of his paper. The specimen, however, is quite a characteristic right duodenal hernia, as can be seen from the photograph. The superior mesenteric artery is seen very distinctly in the anterior margin of the sac.

On closely examining the more or less perfect records of these cases, I find that 7 cases (Klob, Gruber, Gerard-

Marchant, Quenu, Furst, Brösike, 2) may be considered to have had the condition of jejunal adhesion described by Brösike. The remaining 7 cases had no sign of this. We must therefore recognise two varieties of right duodenal hernia: (1) Those in which the fossa exists in association with an adherent jejunum. The length of jejunum fused to the posterior abdominal wall may vary from half an inch up to approximately 4 inches. (2) Those in which the fossa exists in the uppermost portion of the meso-jejunum, close to the duodenum. The jejunum has in these cases a free mesentery from its origin. For the first variety the term 'hernia mesenterico-parietalis para-jejunalis' would be applicable, and for the latter 'hernia mesenterico-parietalis para-duodenalis.'

One fact, which has probably some significance, is that in some cases—Zwaardemaker's, Neumann's, and others—a twisting of the gut, amounting, it is said, to volvulus, has been found at the orifice of the sac. Whether this was present in Dr. Barrs' case I do not remember, but the terrifically sudden onset of the very tight distension would seem to suggest that.

PERIOD OF ONSET OF DUODENAL HERNIA.

With regard to the time of origin of these various forms of internal hernia much doubt exists. Treitz's view was that the development of the sac was delayed until late on in life in most cases, and he considered that there was some connection between profound mental disturbance and the formation of the hernia.

Herniæ are found at all periods of life. So far as I am aware, there is no record of any one having been found in the body of a fœtus. The youngest case is one of Brösike's, that I have previously referred to. The child was fourteen days old. Treitz records one in a girl aged two months.

The existence, or even the possibility, of a congenital hernia has been very often, and with quite unnecessary vigour, denied. It seems to me that all the essentials for the development of a hernia are present during intra-uterine life. Duodenal hernia is, to say the least, very rare, and it could perhaps hardly be expected that, when so few examples are recorded, one should have been found in the fœtus.

The sac, and the orifice bounded by a resistant vessel, and intestine capable of entering the sac, are all present long before birth, and, if present, can surely develop a hernia. Under precisely analogous circumstances occurring in an inguinal hernia we should describe the condition as 'congenital hernia.' Why apply the name to the one and refuse it to the other?

The majority of the cases recorded have occurred in patients who have died of internal strangulation. It is perfectly obvious, from an examination of the bodies in these cases, that such a profound deviation from the normal as exists then must have been the work of years. The hernia is chronic, whether congenital or acquired; the strangulation alone is acute. In some of the smaller cases—found in children—the hernia has been discovered purely by accident. Mr. Shattock's very beautiful specimen is an example of this kind. There is good reason to suppose that, had the child lived, this hernia would have gone on increasing until a sac filling the abdomen had been formed. Then strangulation might have supervened, causing obstruction and death.

DIAGNOSIS.

As a general rule, a duodenal hernia is found accidentally in the post-mortem room. In a few cases—those, namely, of Bordenave, Bryk, Ridge and Hilton, Hauff, Peacock, Zwaardemaker, Quenu, Barrs, Neumann, Brösike—acute intestinal obstruction has been the direct cause of death. This is especially frequent, then, in the form described as right duodenal hernia.

Jonnesco divides all cases into four clinical classes:

1. The hernia is found accidentally on post-mortem examination.
2. Herniæ which have manifested their existence during life by slight digestive troubles.
3. Herniæ which have given rise to chronic intestinal obstruction.
4. Herniæ which have caused acute intestinal obstruction.

This classification is a purely artificial one, and except for the fact that it gives a certain academic completeness, could be best neglected. It is quite possible that a single hernia might fall under each of the four headings, for acute obstruction might supervene upon chronic, and the cause remain unknown till after death.

Physical Signs.—It is an important question, however, to consider whether there are any physical signs by which we are able to predict with a fair degree of accuracy the existence, during life, of these forms of hernia. That such a diagnosis might be possible was, I believe, first suggested in the admirable article by Leichtenstern in Ziemmsen's Cyclopædia in the following words : ' Under favourable circumstances, if the hernia is of notable size, I consider it possible to make a probable diagnosis—not a positive one, but still, one that is based upon reasons. The circumscribed globular distension of the mesogastrium, with retraction of the region corresponding to the colon ; the firm, elastic, spherical lump which can be distinctly felt when the abdominal wall is thin, giving the impression of a large, somewhat movable cyst, and extending from the mesogastrium to the left ; the peculiarity that this well-defined tumour always yields a sonorous note on percussion, and clear intestinal sounds on auscultation, also the presence of hæmorrhoids and the loss of blood from the rectum in consequence of compression of the inferior mesenteric vein—permit, when taken in connection with the subjective troubles indicating chronic disease of the abdominal organs, a probable diagnosis to be made.'

There are three cases which are especially worthy of study in this respect. They are reported by Strazewski, Staudenmayer (the first and only one diagnosed during life), and Barrs. From these it will be seen that there is a certain aggregation of physical signs that should be some help to a diagnosis. The chief sign is, of course, the existence of a localized abdominal swelling. This swelling will have a different position in cases of left and right hernia, but the physical attributes of the mass will be the same in each case.

In Staudenmayer's case the following description is given: ' The onset of symptoms was very acute, the child, aged seven, suddenly crying out, "Oh mother, my belly!" On a first examination the abdomen was tender and tense, but there was nothing to be felt.' This was on April 27. On May 2 (the child being meanwhile treated by opium and enemata) it is noted that 'the abdomen is not generally distended, but in the left hypochondrium there is a circumscribed projection giving an increased sense of resistance. The exact delimitation of the swelling was not possible, as the whole region was tympanitic.' 'On May 4 the tumour had enlarged towards the umbilicus. Behind, the tumour reached to the vertebral column. The swelling is solid and painful. On percussion there are two tympanitic regions—one in the middle, where one sees three intestinal loops running obliquely one above the other, each giving a slightly different percussion note; and another at the sides and below the tumour, which gives a more tympanitic note than the other. On the tumour itself, the note is strikingly tympanitic.'

One feature of this case, which is important, is the development of a large collateral vein on the anterior wall of the abdomen 'between the epigastric and the mammary.'

In Strazewski's case it is reported that 'in the middle of the abdomen, in the region of the umbilicus, there was a tumour, equal in size to a child's head, almost spherical. Firm to the touch, the tumour could be easily depressed; was slightly movable, but not during inspiration, and did not adhere to the posterior abdominal wall. The outline was slightly undulated. To a very slight percussion the sound was dull; on deeper percussion it was hollow and tympanitic.'

A most interesting feature of this tumour was the variation in its size noticed from time to time. The alteration in the magnitude of the tumour, and the aggravation of the symptoms, tallied precisely.

It is specially noted that the hæmorrhoidal veins were very much dilated.

In Barrs' case (right duodenal) the appearance of the abdomen on the post-mortem table was so striking that a drawing (Fig. 22) was at once made. 'The walls were extremely tense from pressure within, which was producing a bulging of the parietes, chiefly or almost entirely involving the lower two-thirds of the abdomen, and so leaving the epigastric region depressed and empty. The abdomen was tympanitic on percussion in all parts. The whole appearance was not much unlike that presented by the abdomen in pregnancy at term.'

The tumour which exists in cases of duodenal hernia may be described, therefore, as having the following attributes:

1. It is limited to a definite region of the abdomen. In left duodenal hernia it lies at first to the left and upper, in right duodenal to the right and lower, part of the abdomen;

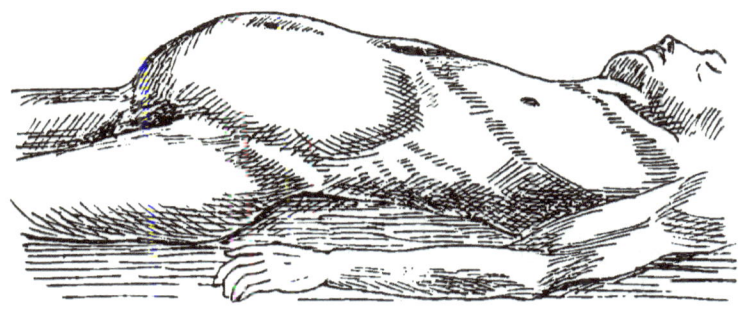

FIG. 22.—APPEARANCE OF THE ABDOMEN IN DR. BARRS' CASE, SHOWING MEDIAN DISTENSION AND FLATNESS IN THE EPIGASTRIC AND COLIC REGIONS.

but in each case spreads finally over almost the whole abdominal cavity. Around the tumour there is an area of depression corresponding to the position of the colon. In size the tumour may vary. It has been described as being of the 'size of a child's head.' In Barrs' case it was 'equal to a nine months' pregnancy.' It is slightly movable, but fixed during respiration.

2. The tumour is marked out distinctly by palpation; on percussion it is always resonant. The degree of resonance varies in different cases, and in different parts of the same tumour. But the striking feature is that the tumour is a *palpable, definite, resonant mass.* In the centre of the tumour, or over its whole surface, may be noticed coils of intestine.

The tumour may bear a very obvious relation to the clinical condition of the patient, becoming more tense and prominent, and very much more tender when the symptoms undergo exacerbation. As the symptoms decline in severity, the tumour becomes less aggressive.

3. On auscultation, distinct gurgling sounds may be heard anywhere in the tumour.

It is an important aid to diagnosis to remember that, owing to the position of the inferior mesenteric vein in the margin of the orifice of the sac of a left duodenal hernia, the radicles of this vein may become enlarged, as in the case of the haemorrhoidal veins, or venous trunks on the anterior abdominal wall may be so increased in size as to form striking features of the case.

So far as the symptoms of the hernia are concerned, there is little to be said. The symptoms may have been so slight that little or no attention was paid to them, or they may have been so sudden as to swiftly strike the patient down when apparently in good health. In the most carefully recorded cases, it is not without some importance to note that a history of chronic slight digestive or intestinal troubles could be obtained. In the recording of future cases, this thorough investigation of the earliest history should be especially attended to.

TREATMENT.

Very little can, or need, be said on this matter. If acute obstruction exists, whatever the diagnosis may be supposed to be, the abdomen will be promptly opened. If a duodenal hernia were found, it would be reduced, and it would further be desirable to divide the neck of the sac—this, of course, between two ligatures, on account of the invariable presence in this position of a large vessel.

Two cases only have proved successful after operation—that of Mr. Tubby in a case of presumably left duodenal hernia, and Neumann's case of the right variety.

CHAPTER III.

THE PERITONEAL FOLDS AND POUCHES IN THE NEIGHBOURHOOD OF THE CÆCUM AND VERMIFORM APPENDIX.

AT the outset of my description of these folds and fossæ, I cannot resist quoting, with entire approval, a remark made by Mr. Treves in his Hunterian Lectures. In his characteristically brisk and forcible phraseology, Mr. Treves remarks that: 'I might be allowed to say that the accounts given of these pouches are somewhat involved, and are frequently contradictory, and, I might venture to add, are also incorrect. Certain fossæ are described as constant that are exceedingly rare. . . . The subject has suffered from a reckless and exuberant nomenclature, etc.' Anyone who has laboriously waded through the not inconsiderable mass of literature upon the subject will cordially re-echo this last sentence.

The same name has by various authors been applied to entirely different fossæ, the term 'ileo-cæcal,' for example, having been applied by one writer or another to every fossa found in this region.

The primary folds determining the existence of fossæ are three in number: An *anterior* raised up by a branch of the ileo-colic artery, which runs over the front aspect of the point of junction of the ileum and colon; a *posterior* raised up by the artery to the appendix; and an *intermediate* fold, which is primarily non-vascular. For this latter fold it is by no means easy to find an exactly appropriate name. Treves proposed the epithet 'bloodless,' until a better should be found. The name, though not strictly accurate, as Treves himself recognised, has a good deal to recommend it. However, it has proved a flaming red rag to Jonnesco and other later authors, who point out, with quite unnecessary emphasis and reiteration, the fact that the fold is by no means devoid of vessels. As this was observed and recorded by Treves in his lectures, the frequent belabouring of the point becomes, apart from its irksomeness, rather amusing.

I must preface my account of the folds by stating that they are seen at their best, in their typical and clearest form, in the young. As the individual increases in years the folds become, from one cause or another, modified to a greater or less degree. I have already referred to this change as occurring in connection with the duodenal fossæ.

A statement, then, as to the precise extent of these folds, based upon an examination of dissecting-room subjects alone —seeing that these are generally middle-aged or old people —cannot be accurate. This fact has lacked appreciation by most authors, and this will, to some degree, explain the anomalies in the several descriptions which have been given.

HISTORY OF THE CÆCAL FOSSÆ.

The first description of any fossa in this region is given, with illustration, by Santorini, in 1775, but until 1834 no further mention is made of it. In this year Huschke described two fossæ bounded by three folds, made evident by traction on the vermiform appendix. The first fold corresponds to the ileo-appendicular, the second to the mesentery of the appendix, and the third, 'or inferior, descends from the mesentery of the appendix towards the external iliac vessels.' Hensing had described the extremities of the right colon and of the left colon as held in position and suspended by two ligaments, which he had named 'ligamentum colicum dextrum' and 'ligamentum colicum inferius.' The former Huschke described under the title 'ligamentum intestini cæci.' Rieux and Engel both have mention of the retro-colic fossæ, the former observer considering that noticed by him as an abnormality. In 1857 Treitz described, in addition to the two fossæ of Huschke, a third or 'sub-cæcal.' ' It lies behind or below the cæcum, and may be called the "sub-cæcal fossa." Sometimes there is but a trivial excavation, at other times there is a sac the length of the finger, the fundus of which lies between the two layers of the ascending mesocolon. The orifice looks downwards and to the front towards the free extremity of the cæcum, which it is necessary to lift up in order to expose the fossa.' Gruber, in 1859, described the last fossa under the uncouth name 'retro-eversio hypogastrica dextra seu inferior dextra.' Luschka, in 1861, gave a fairly accurate account of the fossæ already mentioned, and made a highly important observation as to the causation of the ileo-appendicular fold. He was the first to demonstrate the constant existence in this fold of muscular fibres, continuous on the one hand with the cæcum and on the other with the ileum. He also describes a fold raised up over the termination of the ileum by a branch of the ileo-colic artery. In 1862 Schott recorded one case of his own and one of Widerhofer's, in which the closing of the mouths of cæcal pouches had led to the formation of cysts. In 1862 Luschka described in greater detail the musculature of the ileo-appendicular fold. In 1867 Bochdalek, junior, describes the appendicular artery as passing either in front or behind the ileum; in the former case the mesenteriolum is continuous with the ileo-colic fold.

The best work up to recent years was published in 1868 by Waldeyer, who described four fossæ:

1. Recessus ileo-cæcalis superior, or fossa of Luschka.
2. Recessus ileo-cæcalis inferior: the upper fossa of Huschke.
3. Recessus cæcalis: the lower fossa of Huschke.
4. Recessus sub-cæcalis: the fossa of Treitz.

In 1870 Hartmann, a pupil of Luschka, described three fossæ.

1. Recessus ileo-cæcalis superior: the fossa of Luschka.
2. Recessus ileo-cæcalis media: the upper fossa of Huschke.
3. Recessus ileo-cæcalis infima: not previously described.

In 1885 Treves gave a description of the 'superior' and 'inferior ileo-cæcal fossæ,' and propounded a theory as to the origin of his bloodless fold (the ileo-appendicular fold) which has excited much discussion. For the rest, the observations are meagre.

In 1887 Tuffier, in discussing the subject of hernia of the cæcum, gave a good description of the ' superior ' and ' inferior ligaments of the cæcum,' and of their influence in maintaining the normal position and relations of the cæcum. In 1890 appeared Jonnesco's work, to which I have already made frequent reference. His account is generally accurate, full, and complete, but marred, as all his work is, by an ' exuberant verbosity ' that is the despair of his readers. He describes an ileo-cæcal fossa, an ileo-appendicular fossa, and two retro-cæcal, an internal and external. In 1893, in Poirier's Anatomy, he mentions only one retro-cæcal fossa.

In 1891 Brösike's work appeared. He recognises a recessus ileo-cæcalis superior and inferior, and a recessus retro-cæcalis as frequent and the recessus ileo-cæcalis infima of Hartmann as exceptional. For the fold formed by the downward prolongation of the enteric mesentery he proposed the name ' Plica infra-angularis.' In 1892 Lockwood and Rolleston published an article 'On the Fossæ round the Cæcum,' which I shall so frequently refer to subsequently that no explicit mention is needed now. The most recent work on this subject is by Berry in 1897. This work, though containing nothing novel, is a plain statement of the conditions he considers normal. It is founded largely on Jonnesco's work. As in the latter, a double retro-colic fossa is described.

It is impossible to over-estimate the confusion in nomenclature that has arisen in dealing with this comparatively simple subject. The exuberance of alternative titles is bewildering. In describing each fold or fossa, I have given that name first which I consider most suitable, and I have given in all cases most of the synonyms that have been employed.

THE ILEO-COLIC ARTERY AND ITS BRANCHES.

The ileo-colic artery, as it approaches the angle of junction of the ileum with the ascending colon, gives off as a rule five branches (Fig. 23). The precise mode of origin of these branches may vary within considerable limits. Perhaps the most frequent arrangement is for the vessel to divide into two main trunks, which subsequently split up, the anterior into two, and the posterior into three, branches. The anterior branches are (1) a branch running to the left along the upper border of the ileum, and (2) a branch which continues in the line of the ileo-colic artery over the ileo-colic

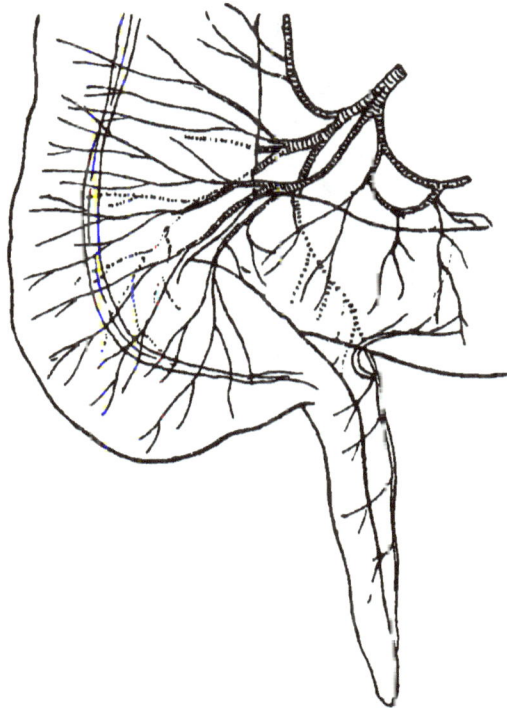

FIG. 23.—DIAGRAM OF THE ILEO-COLIC ARTERY AND ITS BRANCHES.

junction, and gives branches to the cæcum, to the ascending colon, and very much smaller twigs to the anterior surface of the illeum. In a certain number of cases the largest branch of this second vessel is a lateral one, which runs to the right on to the ascending colon, forming in its course a well-defined curve with the concavity directed upwards and to the right.

76 THE CÆCUM AND VERMIFORM APPENDIX

The posterior branches are: (1) A branch running upwards to anastomose with the right colic artery; (2) a branch which runs to the posterior aspect of the angle of junction of the ileum with the colon, distributing branches to the cæcum and colon; and (3) the appendicular artery which runs behind the ileum, in the meso-appendix, to the tip of the vermiform

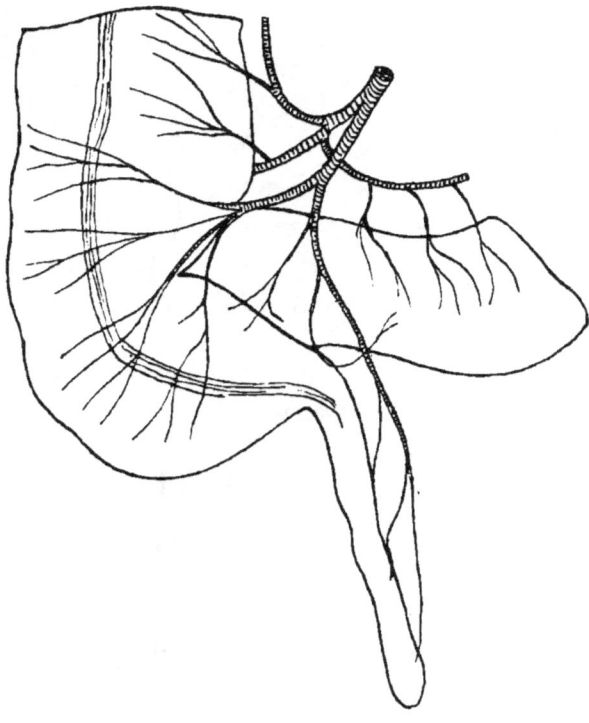

FIG. 24.—DIAGRAM OF THE ILEO-COLIC ARTERY AND ITS BRANCHES WHEN THE APPENDICULAR ARTERY LIES IN FRONT OF THE ILEUM.

process. The chief branch of this last vessel is one which arises at, or very near to, the lower margin of the ileum, and runs with a curve downwards and to the right, and again arches upwards and to the left between the layers of the 'bloodless' fold of Treves near the free edge. The importance of these vessels becomes apparent when we study the folds and fossæ.

THE FOLDS AND FOSSÆ.

The *primary* folds are:

1. The anterior vascular, or ileo-colic fold.
2. The accessory anterior vascular fold.
3. The intermediate, or ileo-appendicular fold.
4. The posterior vascular fold, or meso-appendix.

The fossæ formed by them are:

1. The anterior vascular, or ileo-colic fossa.
2. The accessory anterior vascular fossa.
3. The ileo-appendicular fossa.

In about 5 per cent. of cases there is found to be a third fossa between the termination of the enteric mesentery and the meso-appendix. This, the inferior ileo-cæcal fossa of Hartmann, will be referred to in detail subsequently.

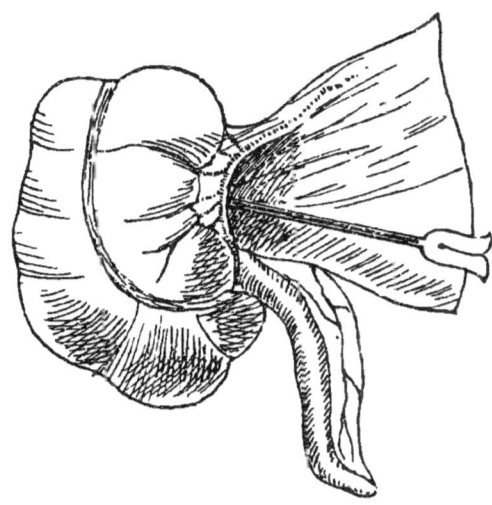

FIG. 25.—THE ANTERIOR VASCULAR (ILEO-COLIC) FOLD AND FOSSA.

The Anterior Vascular Fold—The Ileo-Colic Fold—The Fold of Luschka (*Superior ileo-cæcal fold*, Waldeyer, Hartmann, Treves, Tuffier; *Ileo-colic fold*, Lockwood and Rolleston, Kelynack, Berry; *Superior cæcal fold*, Pérignon; *Mesenterico - cæcal, anterior ileo-cæcal, or pre-ileal*, Jonnesco—Fig. 25).—This fold is raised up by the branch of the ileo-colic artery already referred to, which, continuing the line of direction of the main trunk, runs over the anterior aspect of the ileo-colic junction. The fold is *constant*. In embryos, children, and young adults, it is always well and clearly defined. In the aged and in the obese, it may become very indistinct and flattened out; but, so far as my experience goes, if carefully looked for when the ileum and cæcum are very moderately distended, it will always be found. In nearly 200 bodies that I have examined on this point, I have found it in every case.

The fold is semilunar in shape, having a curved attachment to the anterior layer of the mesentery, the anterior aspect of the ascending colon, and the cæcum down to the root of the appendix. This line of attachment varies in length with the age of the patient. In the embryo and the young, it extends in every case to the appendix. In later years it may end on the colon, just below the level of the upper margin of the ileum, a condition of things which is considered normal by Lockwood and Rolleston. The free edge of the fold containing the vessel looks to the left, and is shorter than the attached margin, representing, as it were, the string of a bow. The fold has two surfaces—one looking to the front and right, and the other, bounding the fossa, to the left and behind. It is thin, sharp, and transparent in youth; thick, dull, and fatty in the aged. In most cases one or, at times, two small lymphatic glands can be seen in its upper part near the attachment to the mesentery.

In some cases the ileo-colic fold is continued on into the meso-appendix, the whole of which is derived from this fold. The artery in the fold then replaces the appendicular artery, and supplies the whole length of the vermiform process. The vascular arrangement will then be that depicted in Fig. 24. In these cases the intermediate (ileo-appendicular) fold joins the posterior surface of the meso-appendix.

In seventeen cases I have met with a distinct fold, and a fossa caused by it raised up by the lateral branch of the ileo-colic artery to which I have previously referred. This fold I propose to call the 'accessory anterior vascular fold' (Fig. 26).

This fold is falciform in shape. Its lower attached margin

is convex, and springs from the anterior aspect of the mesentery (from ½ inch to 1¼ inches above the ileo-colic junction), and from the anterior surface of the ascending colon. The free concave, upward-looking edge contains the lateral branch of the ileo-colic artery, running to supply the front wall of the colon. The fold, when sharply defined, may be more distinct than the ileo-colic fold with which it co-exists. Its surfaces are anterior and posterior, the latter bounding the accessory anterior vascular fossa.

This fold has escaped the observation of all previous writers. I have seen it in seventeen cases quite well defined, both in embryos and in adults. I have photographed some of the examples, and on several occasions I have been able to demonstrate it to others.

The Anterior Vascular Fossa—Fossa of Luschka—Ileo-Colic Fossa (*Superior ileo-cæcal fossa*, Waldeyer, Treves, Hartmann, Tuffier; *Recessus ileo-cæcalis anterior*, Brösike; *Anterior ileo-cæcal or pre-ileal fossa*, Jonnesco; *Ileo-colic fossa*, Lockwood and Rolleston, Kelynack, Berry).—This is a narrow fossa, or chink, situated between the anterior vascular or ileo-colic fold in front, and the enteric mesentery, ileum, and a small portion of the upper and inner part of the cæcum behind. In size and depth the fossa is liable to considerable variation. In the young it is well marked; but in later life, owing to the increase in size of the cæcum, which is chiefly in the transverse direction, and to the invasion of the ileo-colic angle with fat, the fossa may become very small, and even disappear. Externally, it is limited by the attachment of the anterior vascular fold; the orifice of the fossa is directed internally to the left.

When the ileo-colic artery is continued down into the mesentery of the appendix—when, that is, the meso-appendix is derived from, and is continuous with, the ileo-colic fold—the anterior vascular fossa is very considerably increased in size; on section it would then appear to be triangular in form, being bounded in front by the ileo-colic fold and its continuation into the meso-appendix, below by the intermediate non-vascular fold, and behind by the ileum and a small portion of the enteric mesentery. Jonnesco's description of this alteration of the fossa is quite wrong. He confuses the fossa with that situated *behind* the intermediate fold, the ileo-appendicular fossa.

The Accessory Anterior Vascular Fossa (Fig. 26).—This fossa lies between the accessory anterior vascular fold in front, and the anterior surface of the ascending colon and its mesentery behind. Its orifice looks almost directly upwards, with occasionally a slight deviation to the right. In depth

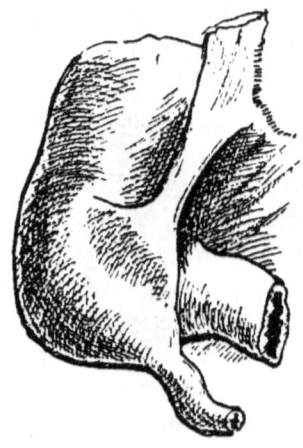

Fig. 26.—The Anterior Vascular Fossa (Ileo-Colic) and the Accessory Anterior Vascular Fossa.

it varies considerably. The deepest fossa I have seen was about 1½ to 1¾ inches from the margin of the fold to the apex near the ileo-colic angle.

The Posterior Vascular Fold—Meso-Appendix (*Mesentery of the vermiform process; mesenteriolum*—Fig. 27).—In order to obtain a good view of this little structure, it is necessary to turn the cæcum and the vermiform appendix upwards. The fold is then seen to spring from the left or posterior layer of the mesentery of the ileum (Fig. 28). I agree with Jonnesco and Berry in thinking that the fold should be described, not as triangular, but as quadrilateral in shape. Its superior border springs from the mesentery along a line which, starting from near the ileo-colic angle, extends upwards and to the left, becoming gradually more distant from the ileum. The right border is attached to the colon on its postero-internal aspect for a short distance, and then to the cæcum. The inferior border is attached to the vermiform appendix, and

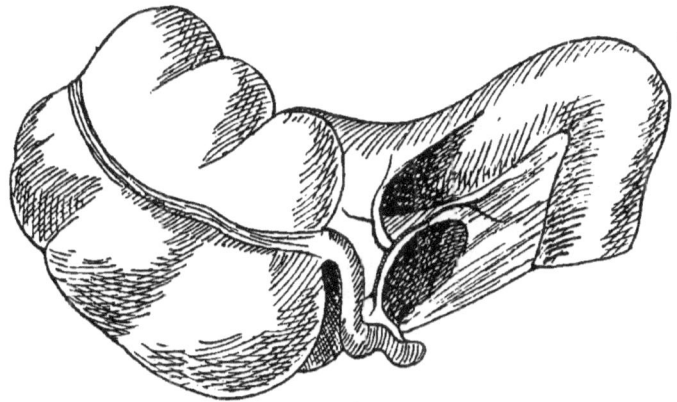

FIG. 27.—THE MESO-APPENDIX AND THE INTERMEDIATE ILEO-APPENDICULAR FOLD AND FOSSA.

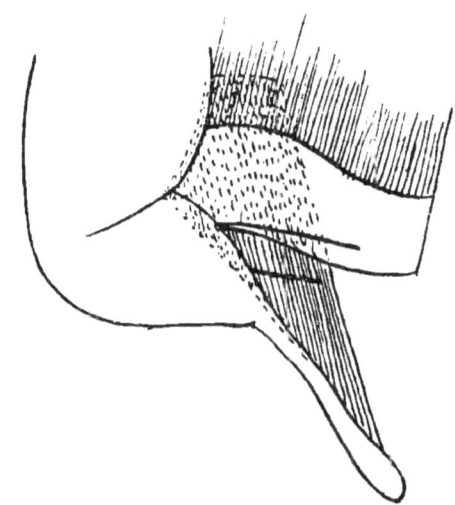

FIG. 28.—DIAGRAM SHOWING THE OUTLINE AND ATTACHMENTS OF THE MESO-APPENDIX AND THE ILEO-APPENDICULAR FOLDS.

the internal or left border is free. There has been much dispute as to the exact length of the attachment of the lower border on to the appendix. Treves, Lockwood and Rolleston,

Fowler and Jonnesco, consider that the fold stops before reaching the end of the appendix. The view I hold coincides with that of Kelynack, Berry and Huntington. It is that the meso-appendix extends throughout the entire length of the tube quite to the very extremity. In some cases the mesentery is continued on to the apex of the process merely as a long, thin, tongue-shaped continuation of the original broad fold. The fold is generally thin and sharply defined, but may, owing to a deposit of fat, become thick and heavy. The left or internal border, which is concave, contains the appendicular artery, a branch of the posterior division of the ileo-colic vessel. The first large branch of the appendicular artery is the recurrent or ileo-appendicular, which will be again referred to. Other branches are given off after this from the lower convex side, and run down to supply the coats of the appendix, and some before it to supply the postero-internal aspect of the cæcum.

The anterior surface of this mesentery is joined by the intermediate or ileo-appendicular fold.

The Ileo-Appendicular Fold—Intermediate Fold (*Superior ileo-cæcal fold*, Waldeyer, Tuffier; *bloodless fold*, Treves; *ileo-cæcal fold*, Lockwood and Rolleston, Kelynack and Berry; *ileo-appendicular fold*, Jonnesco, Juvara—Figs. 27, 28).—Of the many names by which this fold has been described, I consider that invented by Jonnesco, 'ileo-appendicular,' to be decidedly the best. It describes accurately the origin and attachment of the peritoneal fold, and it is so distinctive as to preclude any likelihood of confusion. The fold extends from the lower border of the ileum—that directly opposite the line of the mesenteric attachment—to the anterior surface of the meso-appendix. It is quadrilateral in outline. The upper border is attached to the ileum for an extent which is extremely variable. An average length would be between $1\frac{1}{2}$ to $2\frac{1}{2}$ inches. The lower border extends from the angle formed by the appendix with the cæcum inwards on the anterior surface of the meso-appendix along a line which is almost parallel with the superior border when the appendix is straightened out. Sometimes this line of adhesion is shifted to the appendix itself. Its outer or right border is attached to the inner aspect of the cæcum as far down as the root of the appendix. Its left or inner border is concave to the left and free. This edge contains the recurrent or ileo-appendicular artery, given off almost immediately below the level of the ileum, from the main appendicular artery. From its origin the little vessel runs slightly downwards and outwards in the meso-appendix, and then, turning, it forms an arch with the convexity downwards and to the left as it runs upwards to the ileum between the layers of the ileo-appendicular fold. The arteries are everywhere accompanied by veins. Between the two layers of peritoneum in the fold are also seen some muscular fibres. These were first noticed by Luschka in 1861. They can be very readily seen in the last months of fœtal existence, and in the early years of life. They are continuous with the muscular fibres of the cæcum on the one hand and of the ileum on the other. If the fold be put tightly on the stretch, it will be seen that in the ileo-cæcal angle the fibres are numerous and closely packed, forming quite dense little bundles, which can be shown to be continuous with the longitudinal fibres of the ileum and cæcum.

Further away from the angle the fibres become thinner, scantier, scarcer, and more spread out. Towards the inner end of the fold they become lost. In adults and the aged there is always a deposit of fat in this fold. In the very obese the fat may be quite one-sixth of an inch in thickness, and form a solid slab, filling up the whole fold and obliterating all trace of the muscular bundles. Luschka considered that this fold acted as a regulator between the ileum and the cæcum, keeping a proper and advantageous relative position for these two viscera. By means of this fold the assumption by the ileum of any extraordinary and vicious position is prevented. To the importance of the muscular fibres and vessels in this fold I shall make subsequent reference.

The fold, then, contains arteries, veins, muscle, and fat. It is capable of increasing very considerably in size on account of the fat lying in it; so large may it become that, as Tuffier says, 'it may resemble a miniature omentum.'

The Ileo-Appendicular Fossa (*Recessus ileo-cæcalis*, Luschka; *inferior ileo-cæcal fossa*, Waldeyer, Tarenetzky, Treves, Tuffier; *vermi-ileo-cæcal fossa*, Clado; *ileo-cæcal fossa*, Lockwood and Rolleston, Kelynack and Berry; *inferior cæcal fossa*, Pérignon; *fossa ileo-cæcalis media*, Hartmann; *ileo-appendicular fossa*, Jonnesco and Brösike).—This fossa lies between the ileo-appendicular fold and the mesentery of the vermiform appendix. On section it is triangular in shape. Above it is bounded by the posterior surface of the ileum and the mesentery immediately adjacent to it, in front and

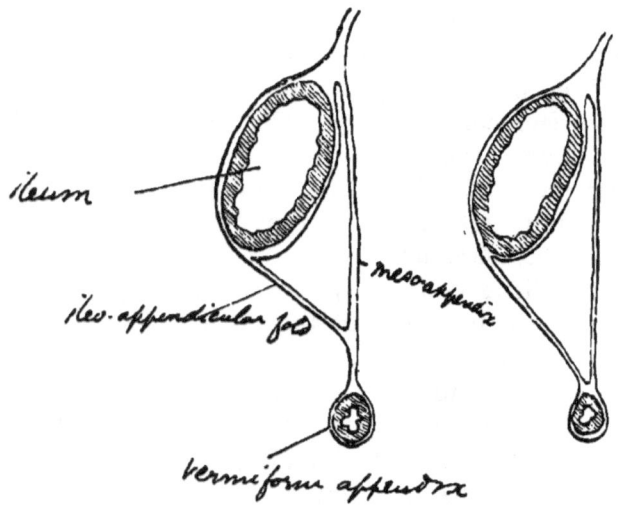

Fig. 29.—Diagrams of the Ileo-Appendicular Fossa.

below by the ileo-appendicular fold, and behind by the upper part of the meso-appendix (Fig. 29). Its anterior superior angle is formed by the line of origin of the ileo-appendicular fold from the ileum; its posterior superior angle by the origin of the meso-appendix from the enteric mesentery: its inferior angle by the junction of the ileo-appendicular fold and the meso-appendix or appendix itself. The size and capacity of this fossa differ very largely, being dependent chiefly on the size of the ileo-appendicular fold. Treves says that the pouch 'will commonly lodge two fingers as far as the first joints.' Sometimes there is a mere chink visible, at other times there is a pocket that would comfortably hold a golf-ball.

Two cases are on record in which it is believed that this fossa has become closed at its mouth, and subsequently dilated to form a cyst. The cases are recorded by Schott. One was seen by Widerhofer in a child eighteen months old; it was full of colloid material, and as large as a walnut. The second contained clear serous fluid, was tightly distended, with thin, tense walls, and was equal in size to an apple.

Fossa Ileo-Cæcalis Infima, Hartmann (*The recessus retro-appendicularis*, Leichtenstern; *the fossa cf Hartmann*, Brösike; *recessus post-iliaci*, Taranetzky).—In some cases the lower attachment of the mesentery to the iliac fossa is prolonged into a sharp fold, termed by Brösike the 'plica infra-angularis.' This corresponds to the 'inferior ligament of the cæcum' of Tuffier. It springs from the ileo-colic angle and from the posterior and inner aspect of the cæcum, and runs backwards to the iliac fossa. Between it and the mesentery of the vermiform appendix there may be found a fossa, the fossa of Hartmann, which is described as being funnel-shaped. Leichtenstern asserts that he has once seen the fossa divided into two by a peritoneal fold, running from the appendix to the parietal peritoneum. I have on a few occasions seen a sort of exaggerated dimple in this position, but never anything worthy of the name of fossa. If a well-defined pouch ever does exist here, it can be of little surgical importance. Leichtenstern believes that Snow's case of hernia, which I shall relate further on, occurred into this pouch, and after carefully thinking the case over I cannot but agree with him. It is, however, the only one of this kind.

Behind the cæcum and ascending colon we not infrequently see a fossa, or more rarely two fossæ, which are due to the secondary adhesion of the ascending colon to the posterior abdominal wall. The extent of this physiological adhesion is capable of great variation, due, as I believe, to the relation which the coils of small intestine bear to the colon. On examining the bodies of fœtuses we find that this relation varies in different subjects and at different ages.

In some it is found that the cæcum and colon, when lying immediately below the liver, are already in contact with the posterior abdominal wall. In others it will be observed that even when the cæcum has reached, or almost reached, the right iliac fossa, there are coils of small intestine between the large gut and the posterior abdominal parietes. In the former class of cases the process of physiological agglutination commences early, and the cæcum, as well as the ascending colon, may be attached to the posterior parietes; in such cases there may be a meso-cæcum, and the cæcum has no peritoneal covering posteriorly. This condition, however, is unusual. In the latter series of cases the secondary adhesion of the colon is delayed until the small intestine coils have withdrawn from their position. In some rare cases such withdrawal never occurs, and the cæcum and colon have then a mesentery in common with the ileum and jejunum. Cases of this kind, as I have already mentioned, are recorded and very beautifully illustrated by Wenzel Gruber.

The influence, therefore, of this process of adhesion upon the fossæ behind the cæcum and colon is a determining one. The presence or absence, the extent and capacity, of the pouches is directly and almost solely dependent upon the activity and degree of the fusion element. I might incidentally remark that it seems to me very probable that the subsequent and eventual position of the vermiform appendix depends also, in no small measure, upon the date and extent of this fusion. If the adhesion takes place early, the appendix is likely to be found in a direction approaching the vertical, with its tip pointing to the left and upwards towards the spleen. If the cæcum remains free until it reaches the iliac fossa, the appendix also will be free and will be pendent, and will be found to hang down into the pelvis. Numerous observations have been made, and carefully prepared statistics published, recording the normal position of the appendix. The appendix can hardly be said to have a single normal position. All the observers, however, with the sole exception of Huntington, completely ignore the question of the amount of posterior adhesion present in the cases observed. To determine this point accurately, and to illustrate the influence of the fusion process on the appendix, it will be necessary in future to observe *firstly* the exact position of the vermiform process, and *secondly* the peritoneal relations of the cæcum and ascending colon. I have little doubt that a constant relationship will be found to exist between the two.

The pouch, or pouches, then, behind the cæcum and colon are *secondary*.

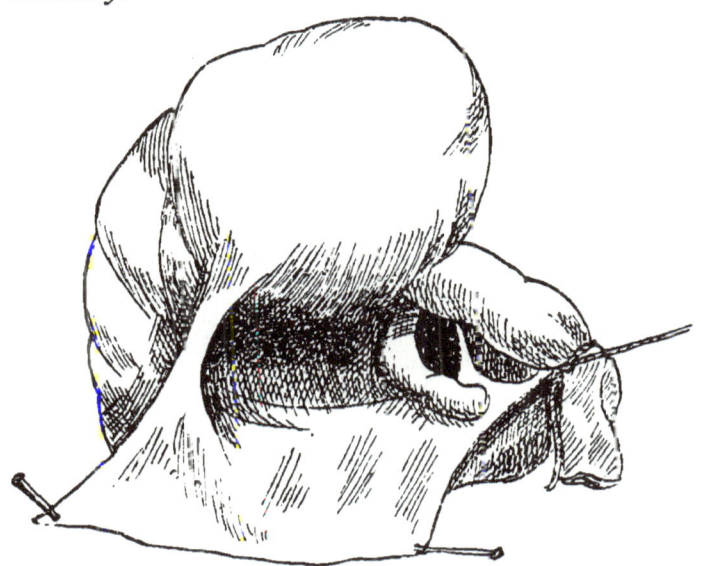

FIG. 30.—THE RETRO-COLIC FOSSA.
The vermiform appendix lies within the fossa.

The Retro-Colic Fossa—Retro-Cæcal Fossa (*Fossa cæcalis*, Huschke, Waldeyer; *fossa post-cæcalis*, Tarenetzky; *Sub-cæcal fossa*, Lockwood and Rolleston; *retro-cæcal fossæ*, Jonnesco; *retro-colic fossæ*, Treves, Berry; *retro-eversio hypogastrica dextra seu inferior dextra*, Gruber; *recessus retro-colicus*, Brösike—Fig. 30).—The term 'retro-colic' is on the whole the most accurate name for this fossa, and the one I shall adopt. In order to see the pouch it is necessary to turn the cæcum upwards. There will then be exposed a fossa of variable size and capacity situated behind the cæcum and the lower part of the ascending colon. In some cases the whole length of the index finger can be comfortably laid in a sort of peritoneal tube which extends upwards to the kidney. In others there may be merely a narrow and shallow dimple that would contain the tip of a lead pencil. Between these two extremes any size may be observed. The fossa is bounded and determined by two peritoneal folds, (*a*) an outer and upper, and (*b*) a lower and inner.

(*a*) **The Parieto-Colic Fold** (*Ligamentum colicum dextrum*, Hensing; *ligamentum intestini cæci*, Huschke; *ligamentum pleuro-colicum*, Langer; *superior ligament of the cæcum*, Tuffier).—This fold is roughly triangular in shape, presenting posterior, anterior, and inferior borders. The posterior border is attached to the abdominal wall, extending from the lower border of the kidney (or even a little higher than this) over the iliac crest to the iliac fossa. The anterior or internal border is attached to the postero-external aspect of the colon, extending not infrequently also on to the cæcum. The lower free border or base, concave in outline, extends from the intestine to the iliac fossa.

The summit or apex of the fold is firmly fixed in the lumbar fossa. To this fold Tuffier, who calls it the 'superior ligament of the cæcum,' attaches great importance as a suspensor and regulator of the position of the cæcum. He describes it as containing tough, strong, shining, fan-shaped fibres, radiating from the apex to the line of insertion on the colon. In addition it carries between its folds several vessels of small size, which anastomose on the one hand with the intestinal vessels and on the other hand with the vessels of the cellular tissue surrounding the kidney. It contains neither lymphatics nor nerves.

(*b*) **The Mesenterico-Parietal Fold** (*Plica ileo-inguinalis*, Engel; *inferior ligament of the cæcum*, Tuffier; *plica infra-angularis*, Brösike).—The term 'mesenterico-parietal,' first suggested by Jonnesco, is on the whole the most suitable and convenient. This fold is, in reality, the insertion of the enteric mesentery into the iliac fossa. It is described by Tuffier as triangular in form. Its base is inserted into the iliac fossa at about the point where the spermatic vessels cross the external iliac artery. This point of insertion is capable of modification. In some cases it is prolonged downwards as far as the inguinal canal in a fold which was described by Treitz as the 'plica genito-enterica.' In other cases it may extend to the pelvic wall, and in women become continuous with the broad ligament. The intestinal border is attached to the small intestine and to the postero-internal aspect of the cæcum and ascending colon. Its free edge is concave, and looks downwards and to the right.

In some cases—such as that described by Langer—these two folds, parieto-colic and mesenterico-parietal, may be continued downwards and coalesce in the formation in the iliac fossa of a falciform fold. In such a case the fossa, bounded below by this fold, would be strictly retro-cæcal. The retro-colic fossa, then, is bounded: in front by the posterior aspect of the ascending colon, and sometimes a portion, or the whole, of the posterior surface of the cæcum; behind by the peritoneum of the iliac fossa; to the right by the parieto-colic fold; and to the left by the mesenterico-parietal fold. Its orifice looks downwards, and into it the vermiform appendix may enter.

In some cases two fossæ are found in this situation, and this condition is looked upon as normal by Jonnesco and Berry. The latter author gives a very clear account of his view, which is to some extent based upon Jonnesco's observations. He describes three folds and two fossæ. The folds are:

1. External parieto-colic (my parieto-colic fold).
2. Internal parieto-colic.
3. Mesenterico-parietal fold.

1 and 2 are the outer and inner layers of the ascending mesocolon. Between 1 and 2 lies the outer retro-colic fossa, and between 2 and 3 the inner retro-colic fossa. Berry himself, however, only found both fossæ present in two cases out of twenty. The arrangement, therefore, can hardly be called normal. I have examined close upon 200 bodies, and my opinion very decidedly is that when any peritoneal pouch is here present it is most commonly single, and bounded and

limited in the manner I have described. Two fossæ result from the very occasional division of the original fossa.

Fossa Iliaco-Subfascialis (*Sub-cæcal or iliac fossa*, Jonnesco; *fossa infra-cæcalis*, Leichtenstern).—The fossa of Biesiadecki. This fossa, which is of some surgical importance, has entirely escaped recognition and description by English authors. It is situated about the middle of the iliac fossa, and in size varies between a small, almost imperceptible transverse slit, and a large fossa with a wide elliptical mouth, measuring $1\frac{1}{2}$ to 2 inches in diameter. The orifice is directed upwards, and is bounded in front by a more or less well-defined fold, the inner extremity of which is directed upwards over the psoas towards the root of the mesentery, and the outer extends towards the iliac crest. It was shown by Biesiadecki that an examination of the iliac fascia elicited the fact that in the upper half of the fossa the fascia was lax, movable, and loosely bound down, whereas in the lower half the fascia was tense, taut, and more firmly fixed. Tarenetzky observed that not infrequently the junction of the two was acutely defined by a sharp, upwardly concave fold. The fossa iliaco-subfascialis, then, is a hernial protrusion of the peritoneum, so to speak, behind this sharp band. Tarenetzky asserts that the fossa may exist on the left side as well as the right, and that it is capable of holding the cæcum, colon, or portions of small intestine.

When the psoas parvus is present, there is not infrequently a peritoneal groove between this muscle and the psoas magnus. This groove has been described as capable of development into a fossa. This is not unlikely, as a hernia described by Wagner was contained in a pouch in this situation. I have myself never seen anything more, however, than the peritoneal groove referred to.

GENESIS OF THE FOLDS AND FOSSÆ.

It was first demonstrated by Waldeyer, and his description has since been universally accepted, that the anterior and posterior vascular folds, the ileo-colic fold, and the meso-appendix, owed their origin to the lifting up of a peritoneal leaf by each of the vessels running from the ileo-colic artery to the cæcum and appendix. The folds contain these arteries at their free edges, and the extent and development of the two folds are entirely and solely dependent upon the vessels. They are, in fact, *vascular* folds. The ileo-appendicular fold has, however, given rise to much discussion, and even yet no completely satisfactory or universally acknowledged explanation has been given of its origin. A reference to its comparative anatomy is exceedingly interesting, as Huntington has pointed out. What may be taken as the most simple and primitive condition of the three primary folds is well exemplified in the black-handed spider monkey, *Ateles ater*. Here the anterior and posterior vascular folds are nearly equally developed; in each of them is a vessel, a branch of the ileo-colic artery. Between the two vascular folds is seen a large, bold peritoneal reduplication—the intermediate or ileo-appendicular fold. It is quite separate from the two vascular folds, though lying nearer to the dorsal than the ventral. In the cæcum of *Mycetes fuscus*, the brown howler monkey of Brazil, the anterior vascular fold is well defined. The posterior vascular fold is extremely short; it blends almost immediately with the intermediate fold, which is of good size. In *Cercopithecus sabræus*, the African green monkey, the arrangement is as follows: The anterior and posterior vascular folds are reduced to a minimum, being mere ridges of peritoneum containing fatty deposits resembling appendices epiploicæ. The anterior vessel is small and quite insignificant, supplying only the front of the ileo-colic junction. The dorsal vessel is large, and supplies the whole of the posterior surface and apex of the cæcum. The intermediate fold is well developed, and lies nearer the dorsal than the ventral artery. Now, Huntington points out that in 'cercopithecus the dorsal aspect of the ascending colon is adherent to the posterior parietal peritoneum down to the iliac region and the beginning of the cæcum, whereas in ateles and mycetes the entire cæcum as well as the ascending colon appear free and non-adherent to the posterior abdominal parietes.' 'The facts would seem to point to the conclusion that in the adhesion of the colic tube to the parietal peritoneum the posterior ileo-colic branches find an element favourable to their more complete development and extension, replacing in part or entirely the anterior artery, which ceases its function below the level of the ileo-colic junction. It is possible that the adhesion and consequent fixation of the posterior-colic wall may afford this advantage to the posterior vessel, whereas the greater mobility and the alternating conditions of distension and contraction, with variations of intra-cæcal pressure from contents, may operate unfavourably upon the development of the anterior vessel.'

Treves, from a study of the comparative anatomy of the folds, has come to the conclusion that the intermediate fold, the 'bloodless' fold, is the true mesentery of the appendix, the meso-appendix being a 'substituted' mesentery. He says: 'The simple cæca of most of the lower animals represent both the cæcum and appendix of the highest mammal. In such animals as have a prominent cæcum it will be noticed that a well-marked fold of peritoneum passes to it from the ileum. The subject may be here simplified by selecting the cæcum of some one animal (and I have arbitrarily selected the kangaroo) as a basis for the description of this very general fold. The fold always passes from that margin of the ileum that is most remote from the attachment of the mesentery to that border of the cæcum that is nearest to the small intestine. It is a thin layer of peritoneum, with a well-defined concave margin, and is singularly free from visible bloodvessels. It is the true mesentery of the cæcum, it is continuous over the ileum with the mesentery of that bowel, and it is evident that it has been derived from the latter membrane by the budding out and growth of the caput coli. As this diverticulum has developed it has carried a part of the common serous investment of the intestine with it. It has nothing to do with conveying blood to the cæcum.' Blood is carried to the cæcum by the vessels in the anterior and posterior vascular folds. 'Now, on turning to the human cæcum, it will be seen that the anterior vascular fold exists as the plica that forms the superior ileo-cæcal fossa (that one which I have called "ileo-colic"). The posterior vascular fold, with its distinct bloodvessel, exists in man as the mesentery of the appendix, while the fold in the human subject that has been termed the "bloodless fold" persists as the remains of the true mesentery of the cæcum and the appendix. The human appendicular mesentery is a substituted mesentery. The true serous fold of that process is represented by the non-vascular plica that runs from the surface of the ileum to the substituted mesentery of the appendix.'

Lockwood and Rolleston say: 'As regards the origin of the ileo-cæcal (*i.e.*, ileo-appendicular) fold, our investigations incline us to think with Mr. Treves that it was originally developed to carry bloodvessels to the cæcum and appendix, but that it has been replaced by the meso-appendix, which affords a shorter and more convenient route. Thus, the ileo-cæcal (ileo-appendicular) fold would correspond to, and be the fellow of, the ileo-colic fold, which, it may be remembered, also carried vessels to the cæcum and appendix, one set passing over the ileum, the other under.'

In discussing this point, Berry says: 'Jonnesco holds that the meso-appendix is the true appendicular mesentery, and that the ileo-colic and ileo-appendicular folds are the mesenteries of the cæcum. That the meso-appendix is not, as Treves would have us believe, a substituted mesentery, says Jonnesco, is proved by the fact that the ileo-cæcal fold is the only one which is ever found wanting. Whilst the writer's statistics do not confirm Jonnesco, they do prove that the meso-appendix is the only constant fold, and the constancy of this mesentery is a fact accepted by almost every author. Arguing from this fact, it would appear that the appendix is gradually replacing the cæcum in functional activity. Such a theory is supported by the facts concerning the peri-cæcal folds; the meso-appendix is the largest, the most constant, the most vascular of the three, hence it is presumably concerned in the more functionally active of the two viscera, etc.' In any case, the facts emphasize the probability of the ileo-colic and ileo-appendicular folds being true cæcal mesenteries, primary and subsidiary respectively, and the meso-appendix the true appendicular mesentery.

A quite different view as to the genesis of the ileo-appendicular fold was given by Luschka. This authority first described the presence and course of bands of muscular fibres contained within the fold. His pupil, Hartmann, suggested that this plica was due to the raising up of the peritoneum by the muscle fibres, which were pulled away, so to speak, from the band of muscular tissue running across the inferior ileo-cæcal angle. Toldt, in 1879, expounded this theory more fully. He says: 'The ileo-appendicular fold has a significance quite other than that of the ileo-colic and meso-appendix. The fact that it does not contain large vessels, but bundles of muscular fibres, which I have found at the end of the fifth month of intra-uterine life (the ileo-colic fold and the meso-appendix, I may here state, appear at the fourth month), and that there exists a union between these fibres and the muscular coat of the intestine, shows that the ileo-appendicular fold is a portion of the peritoneal investment detached from the cæcum. The fold so formed increases in size in proportion to the amount of separation of the ileum from the appendix.'

According to the theory expressed by these authors, then, the fold is *muscular* in origin.

I do not consider that either of these theories is completely satisfactory, and in this belief I am ranging myself alongside both Brösike and Jonnesco. The theory of Treves has, to my mind, no evidence to support it; it is wholly untrue. The theory of Luschka, Hartmann, and Toldt is partially true only.

If an embryo of the fourth month be examined, it will be found that at the point of budding, where the cæcum is developing, an artery (the ileo-colic) supplies two branches to the bud, one anterior, the other posterior. These two vessels lie on the surface of the gut, immediately beneath the layers of the peritoneum. As the cæcal bud increases in size, sprouting away from the mesenteric attachment, it will drag its vessels with it; but the cæcal growth is more rapid than the vascular. The result is that the vessels seek a short path, and run straight to their destination, instead of following the outline of the gut. In doing so they pull up and drag upon the peritoneum in their neighbourhood, and so lead to the formation of two distinct plicæ, the anterior and posterior vascular folds already referred to. At the end of the fifth month, when the cæcal bud is easily recognisable, there is seen in between the ileum and the cæcum the intermediate fold already developed, and containing between its layers the bundles of muscle fibre that I have described. Now, from the posterior or dorsal vessel, running in the posterior vascular fold, a branch is given off, which, running in a curved direction, mounts upwards eventually to the ileum. This is the ileo-appendicular artery, which lies in the free edge of the ileo-appendicular fold. The later development of this fold then, it would seem, depends upon the vessel in its free margin. This theory, therefore, looks upon the ileo-appendicular fold as of a twin origin; it is a compound fold. Primarily, and in the first instance, it is muscular, dependent upon the ileo-appendicular muscle; later its development is modified by and attributable to the ileo-appendicular artery, the recurrent branch of the main appendicular vessel. This being the case, the ileo-appendicular fold is, in part, at least, secondary to and dependent upon the posterior vascular fold, the meso-appendix. It is the last fold to appear in the embryo, less constant than the meso-appendix, and receives its vessel (upon which it to some extent depends for its existence) from the posterior vascular fold. It cannot therefore be the primitive mesentery of the cæcum.

With regard to the genesis of the retro-colic fossæ, I have already remarked that they are *secondary*, and are dependent upon the coalescence, sometimes wanting, of the posterior surface of the ascending colon, and sometimes, though very rarely, of the cæcum, to the posterior wall of the abdomen. If the cæcum and ascending colon are free, and covered on their posterior surfaces by peritoneum, these secondary fossæ are absent. But whatever the position of the cæcum, normal or abnormal, the three primary folds and the two fossæ caused by them are present in a more or less obvious condition. Treitz, in his work already alluded to, gives expression to his belief that the retro-colic fossa, and on the left side the intersigmoid fossa, depend for their existence upon the descent of the testicle or the ovary. The mesorchium was, he asserted, united to the serous covering of the cæcum. During the descent of the testicle the plica genito-enterica pulled on the cæcum, causing its descent, and raising up a peritoneal fold, which became the boundary of the subcæcal fossa. His view, however, has been so completely discussed and negatived by Waldeyer that nothing is left for any later author to debate. And the fact that the fossæ have been seen in cases of retentio abdominalis testis gives the final answer to Treitz's theories, which, it is interesting to remember, were without question accepted by Gruber. Waldeyer's own theory was based on an incomplete and erroneous view of the cæcal transition. He asserts that the cæcum continues its descent after the ascending colon has become fixed, and thereby raises up by traction peritoneal folds, which bound a 'primary' fossa. Lockwood and Rolleston practically restate in slightly modified terms the views of Treitz and Gruber. The theory of Toldt, however, that these folds and pouches are secondary, must now, I think, receive general acceptance.

PERICÆCAL HERNIA.

So far as I am aware—and I have, I think, exhaustively studied the literature of this subject—there are no cases on record which can be considered as hernial protrusions into either the *ileo-colic fossa* or the accessory anterior vascular fossa. The fossæ are only of anatomical interest. They have no pathology.

With regard to the **Ileo-appendicular Fossa.**

This fossa as a general rule is small, and the peritoneal folds binding it are lax and in fairly close relationship to one another. A hernia into this pouch is likely therefore to be unusual. If by any process of physiological or pathological adhesion the vermiform process becomes fixed in the iliac fossa, then a distension and a dragging of the ileum would cause the mouth of the pouch to gape. Similarly, a bulky filling of the cæcum, and a simultaneous tugging on the lower part of the ileum, would render the ileo-appendicular fold and the meso-appendix taut, and thereby make wide the orifice of this sac. Under such or similar circumstances a portion of the small intestine might enter the fossa, and there become lodged and perhaps strangled.

The only cases, however, that I have been able to discover of hernia of this variety, where small intestine lay in the sac, are:

   1. Tuffier's case.
   2. Specimen in the Musée Dupuytren.
   3. Little's case.
   4. Partridge's case.

Cases 1 and 2 are referred to by both Jonnesco and Brösike. The third case, Little's, has not been noticed by either of these authorities. It is, however, the best authenticated, and the narration of it is illustrated by two highly-instructive figures. Case 4 has also been overlooked.

CASE 1. *Tuffier's Case.*—The record of this is very unsatisfactory: 'Among a large number of bodies that I have examined, I have had the good fortune to discover this hernia (ileo-appendicular) in its most marked form. The subject was a man fifty years of age, very stout. An intestinal loop, which unrolled measured 8 centimetres, was contained in this pouch, which was very dilated. The fossa was enlarged upwards and backwards; its base corresponded to the postero-inferior part of the cæcum, but there was no sign of a neck, or of strangulation; the bowel entered and left the sac without difficulty.'

We must accept this case as an ileo-appendicular hernia, but one must protest against the poverty and incompleteness of the description of so important a case.

CASE 2. *Case in the Musée Dupuytren.*—A reference to this specimen (*pièce de Michon*) is made by Tuffier, who considers it a true specimen of ileo-appendicular hernia; but Jonnesco, who has examined the specimen, remarks that 'it is not very convincing.'

CASE 3. *Internal Strangulation—Anatomy of the Vermiform Appendix*, Dr. T. E. Little (Fig. 31).—'The specimen on the table consists of the terminal portion of the small, and the commencement of the large, intestine, with their peritoneal attachments. It was removed from the body of a man aged sixty, of powerful frame of body, who had enjoyed excellent health up to the moment of the fatal attack, nine days after the first evidence of which he died, from symptoms which may, in brief, be described as those of unrelieved strangulated hernia.

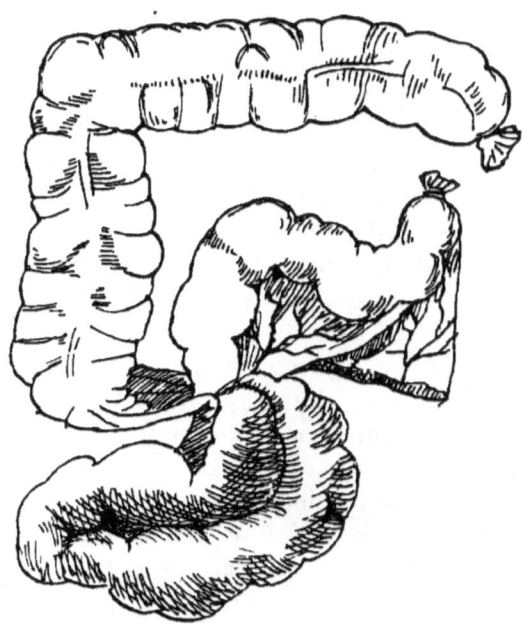

Fig. 31.—Ileo-Appendicular Hernia. (Little's Case.)

'On opening the body all the organs examined were found to be perfectly healthy, except those concerned in the lesion under observation.

'There was no general peritonitis, and even in the region of the strangulated gut but a very small amount of lymph was to be seen between the intestinal folds.

'From a point near the tip of the vermiform appendix a narrow but strong whitish band is seen passing to an attachment into the front of the ileum at a distance of about 2 inches from the termination of the latter gut, and through the opening left between this cord, the appendix itself and its attachments, a large loop (16 or 18 inches in length) of that part of the ileum immediately above the attachment of the band alluded to has become prolapsed, and is tightly constricted—so tightly that in the recent specimen a narrow probe was with difficulty passed between the constriction and the intestine. The piece of gut strangulated is of deep-brown colour, is much distended, and is in a condition of incipient gangrene, the peritoneum stripping off it in most places under the mere touch of the finger.

'In endeavouring to interpret these post-mortem phenomena, it might seem as if the obstruction resulted from an abnormal band of adhesion, connecting the vermiform process and the ileum; but on looking more closely to the particulars of the case, and the appearances met with, there seem to be many things against this solution of the matter. No pathological trace of peritonitis existed in the abdominal cavity, nor was there any other appearance of adhesion discoverable in the neighbouring or any of the other regions of the abdomen; the vermiform appendix itself, and the part of the ileum to which the band is attached, are both perfectly healthy; no account of any antecedent attack of peritonitis, or of the occurrence of any important abdominal affection, appears in the history of the patient's previous health; the peritoneum is carried over the constricting band uninterruptedly, just as over the neighbouring organs; and, again, the fact that the band is attached to the side and not to the tip of the vermiform appendix is consistent with the explanation to be given.'

Dr. Little then discusses, with perfect accuracy, the anatomy of the appendix, its mesentery, and the ileo-appendicular fold, and concludes that the case is one of hernia between these two folds, and that the constricting band 'is not a pathological product, but a normal anatomical structure.'

The report of this case is a model of what such descriptions should be, and is so full and complete, and the accompanying drawings are so convincing, that we may without hesitation accept the case as one of ileo-appendicular hernia.

CASE 4. *Internal Strangulation of the End of the Small*

Intestine (Ileum), produced by its Passage through an Aperture in the Vermiform Appendix, by Mr. Partridge.—A maidservant, aged twenty-six, died after five days' illness of acute obstruction. The post-mortem examination showed the small intestines greatly distended, the large bowel quite empty, slight traces of peritonitis. A knuckle of the ileum, immediately above its termination, was found strangulated and much congested, in consequence of having passed through, and become impacted in, a hole or interspace in the mesentery of the vermiform appendix. The strangulated portion of the bowel was of a deep-red colour, and some recent lymph was effused upon its peritoneal surface, as well as upon the surface of the adjacent parts.' [The specimen from this case cannot be found.]

This account is very paltry, but is, I think, capable of only one explanation. The condition is strictly comparable to the preceding one of Little's, and must therefore be accepted as authentic.

The cases mentioned above are, as I have stated, examples of the hernial intrusion of small intestine into the ileo-appendicular fossa. In addition to these, several examples have been incidentally recorded from time to time of hernia of the vermiform process into this pouch. This condition I believe to be not very unusual. I have seen from time to time many specimens of it. Lockwood, in the 'Pathological Society's Transactions,' in discussing the subject of retro-peritoneal hernia of the vermiform appendix, says that 'it may occur into either the subcæcal or ileo-cæcal fossæ; it may be partial or complete; the mouth of the fossa may be completely closed.'

In the majority of examples that I have examined the appendix lay free and unattached in the fossa, or adherent, at the most, by very flimsy filaments of lymph. In some, however, the appendix was firmly and inseparably soldered to the walls of the sac. I have—though rarely—seen the appendix contained within the cavity, when the mouth of the pouch was completely closed up. Under these circumstances it may appear, after a more than cursory examination, that the appendix is absent. A careful search will reveal the true condition of affairs. Absence of the appendix, described by some authors, must be very exceptional. I have never met with a case.

The clinical importance of hernia of the vermiform process into this fossa or a retro-colic fossa will be dealt with subsequently.

It will be important in any future case to observe the relationship of the appendicular and ileo-appendicular arteries to the orifice of the sac. If the appendicular artery is behind the mouth, the hernia will have developed in the ileo-appendicular fossa. If the artery lies in front, the intestine will lie in the fossa of Hartmann—provided, of course, that the normal position of the parts is adhered to.

HERNIA INTO THE FOSSA OF HARTMANN.

A Case of Strangulation of the Ileum in an Aperture in the Mesentery, by John Snow, M.D.—'The subject of this case was a lady, aged twenty-four. When in the eighth month of pregnancy she was seized with severe pain in the belly, of an intermitting character, with sickness and vomiting. She thought labour was coming on, but there was no dilatation of the os uteri. The symptoms throughout her illness were those usually arising from some mechanical obstruction in the bowels, and, in spite of all the remedies employed, they continued with more or less severity until her death, which took place on the fourth day.

'An examination of the body was made twenty-four hours after death, and the morbid appearances are fully detailed. On examining the preparation which was on the table, the vermiform appendix is found enclosed within a double layer of peritoneum, which forms a kind of broad ligament, which is attached above to the cæcum and ileum, and externally and inferiorly to the iliac fossa and brim of the pelvis. On the outer side of the vermiform appendix there is an aperture in this membrane with defined edges, through which the thumb can be passed, and behind the portion of it which extends with a curve from the appendix to the ileum there is a pouch into which a finger can be passed for about two inches. The thin membrane passing across from the vermiform appendix to the ileum and leaving the aperture through which the aperture [*sic*—this should surely read 'hernia'] forms an extension of the above-named curve. The author remarks that there are many cases on record of strangulation of the bowel from adhesion of the vermiform appendix with neighbouring parts; but the appearance of the membrane in this case, the absence of the evidence of old inflammation, and the circumstance that the membranous band appears to be a natural continuation of a larger fold, leads him to consider it as a congenital production of peritoneum, leaving an aperture on the inner side of the appendix vermiformis similar to the one seen on its outer side.'

This account is very obscurely worded, and is written in complete ignorance of the normal anatomy of the parts. I think, however, that the only reasonable view to take of the case is to regard it as a hernia into the fossa of Hartmann.

HERNIA INTO THE RETRO-COLIC FOSSA.

Treitz, in discussing the cases of hernia into the subcæcal (as he termed it) fossa, refers to two examples only. The first is the case of Snow's—already reproduced—which I have shown is in all probability an example of hernia into the fossa of Hartmann, and Wagner's, which, although accepted by Jonnesco and other writers, I unhesitatingly refuse as an authentic example. In asking the question why this form of hernia was so rare, Treitz suggested as answers:

1. Because the orifice of the sac looks downwards, and therefore the intrusion of the gut is to some extent prohibited by reason of their weight.

2. Because the orifice of the sac is not resistant, and does not contain any vessel.

Jonnesco criticises these remarks in a most unfortunate manner. He asserts:

1. That the hernia is not very rare.
2. That the orifice of the sac is not devoid of resistance.

3. That, not infrequently, he has met with intestinal loops between the cæcum and the posterior abdominal wall—loops which were capable, under great abdominal pressure, of being pushed up into the retro-colic pouch.

In answer I would venture to affirm :

1. That retro-colic hernia, as I hope to show, is exceedingly rare.

2. That in the normal condition—that is, in the absence of peri-appendicitis, etc.—the greater part of the mouth of the fossa is quite devoid of resistance.

3. Intra-abdominal pressure, produced in the manner suggested, is equalized throughout the whole abdominal cavity, and there is no reason to suppose, but on the contrary every reason to negative, any selective effect such as is here suggested.

Seeing that the cases recorded as retro-colic hernia, and accepted by most authors, including Jonnesco, are to my mind by no means to be unhesitatingly accepted, I propose to pass them briefly in review.

These cases are: 1 by Fages, 1 by Wagner, 1 by Parise, 3 by Rieux, 1 by Engel, 1 by Klebs, 1 by Moxon, 1 by Josse, 1 by C. Furst.

Case related by Fages.—This was a hernia in a monorchid. The right side of the scrotum had always been empty. The patient died of obstruction. On examining the body after death, it was found that a hernial loop was contained within a 'special sac formed by the peritoneum, situated on the anterior and middle portions of the psoas, and on the right side of the rectum.' The testicle and the epididymis lay at the postero-inferior portion of the sac. Fages believed that the hernia lay in the tunica vaginalis. Duchaussoy, in commenting upon the description, suggested that the case was an example of hernia inguinalis intra-iliaca. Broca considered it to be a congenital hernia in association with a retained testicle. Exactly what form of hernia it was I am not prepared to say, but it most certainly was not retro-colic.

There is not a word in Fages' account of any sort of relationship with the cæcum or colon. On the whole, I am inclined to accept the explanation of Broca.

Case related by Wagner.—This occurred in a man thirty-four years of age. Death from obstruction.

The strangulated gut was about 3 inches in length, and lay in a fossa which was placed 'about 7 lines below the right inguinal ring on the iliacus muscle; it extended upwards and outwards from the inner and anterior border of the psoas, and was bounded by a ring about 1 inch in diameter.'

This description, which agrees with the illustration, does not tally with any well-recognised fossa. Brösike states that on two occasions he has found in very thin people a small fossa lying transversely between the psoas magnus and the psoas parvus in the position I have previously described. This fossa would be in very much the same position as Wagner's hernial sac, but it is not stated that the tendon of the psoas parvus lay in the anterior margin of the sac, as would inevitably be the case if a hernial protrusion lay in Brösike's fossa. So that it is a matter of uncertainty as to what precise form of hernia this is, but the fact of its lying behind the peritoneum of the iliac fossa proves beyond the possibility of doubt that it is not retro-colic.

Case related by Parise. — Male, aged thirty-four. 'The hernial sac occupied the right iliac fossa, lay underneath the iliac fascia, and was covered above and on the inner side by the cæcum. Near its neck the sac sent a prolongation down the inguinal canal.' The patient had a retained testicle on the same side.

This case has given rise to considerable discussion, and various opinions have been expressed by Parise, Cruveilhier, Gosselin, and others.

Read in the light of our present knowledge, there can, I think, be little doubt that the hernia is one of the variety described by Krönlein as 'hernia inguinalis intra-iliaca.' It most decidedly is not retro-colic.

Three Cases recorded by Rieux: First Case.—Woman, aged forty-two. Death from obstruction.

'Eight centimetres of small intestine penetrated an abnormal cavity underneath the cæcum. This cavity terminates in a cul-de-sac measuring 7 centimetres in a transverse direction—that is, in depth. It is entirely covered on its superior as well as inferior aspects by a peritoneal fold in all respects similar to that which covers the superior face of the cæcum.

Around the orifice of entry into this sac there is a thickening of the cellular tissue (sub-peritoneal), causing a circular elevation of the peritoneum. If traction is exerted upon the peritoneum a little distance away, this circular elevation is thrown into bands, which completely close the orifice of the sac as with a purse-string suture.'

The meaning of this description is not very clear. Most probably it argues of peritonitis and the formation by lymph and adhesions of an abnormal pouch in the close neighbourhood of the cæcum. I think that we must allow the case to go undiagnosed. The hernia probably is not retrocolic.

Second Case.—Male, aged forty-four. Death from obstruction.

'The intestinal distension continued to the level of the ileo-cæcal valve. At this point I found the last portion of the small intestine placed underneath the cæcum, and I drew out about 5 centimetres of collapsed gut. It was caught in a sort of cavity bounded by peritoneum, closed below by a tight peritoneal band, and in part by the cæcum. The cavity could contain about half the length of the little finger.'

This record, again, is unsatisfactory; the description is bald and devoid of that exactness which would enable us to accurately classify it. The most that can be said is that it is not improbably a case of retro-colic hernia.

Third Case.—Infant of fifteen months. Death from acute pneumonia.

'Four or five centimetres of small intestine penetrated into an abnormal cavity beneath the cæcum, about 4 centimetres in depth, entirely lined by peritoneum; the aperture of entry was bounded by two slight ridges of peritoneum.

'There was no sign of any obstruction to the passage of food along the canal.'

That is all. The description lacks completeness and detail, and, as of the second case, it can only be, without improbability, accepted as a retro-colic hernia.

Case related by Engel.—Soldier, aged thirty-one. Death from pneumonia.

The following description is given: 'The cæcal pouch was dilated so as to contain the small intestine with the exception of the upper portion of the jejunum and the lower portion of the ileum. The orifice of the sac admitted two fingers. As this sac was developed wholly in the right half of the abdomen, the cæcum was pushed above and to the left of the umbilicus, and the colon and sigmoid flexure were pressed to the left. The intestine was distended with gas, but could be removed from the sac quite easily, and could be freely replaced.' This description is meagre and insufficient. Engel describes it as a case of retro-cæcal hernia, and we have nothing more than his word, unsupported, to rely upon. No facts are given upon which we can form a judgment for ourselves. The case cannot be unhesitatingly accepted, and its true nature must remain a matter of doubt. Leichtenstern affirms that the hernia occurred into the fossa iliaco-subfascialis.

Case of Klebs.—Klebs relates in his work, with unfortunate brevity, the case of a young man in whom death resulted from a snaring of a portion of the small intestine which lay beneath the cæcum. There is no mention of any sac containing the strangulated portion of the bowel, and it is not unlikely that the retro-cæcal position of the strangled segment of the gut was accidental, and independent of the occluding cause.

Case of Moxon, related by Pye-Smith.—' In a case to which Dr. Moxon kindly called my attention a few months ago I found several feet of the latter end of the ileum contained in a large and well-marked retro-peritoneal sub-cæcal pouch. The person in whose body this hernia was discovered had exhibited no symptoms of intestinal obstruction during life, and the incarcerated coils of gut, which were easily removed, showed no trace of inflammation, congestion, or adhesion to the sac. The mesentery attached to the ruptured intestine was thick from sub-peritoneal fat, and formed a bulky folded border at the entrance to the sac. This case I have examined in the Guy's Museum. It is Specimen 1084, and is clearly one of right duodenal hernia, and as such I have already counted it.

Case of Josse.—A young man twenty-four to twenty-six years of age.

On the left side there was a large irreducible inguinal hernia, at the bottom of which was felt a mass of the size and consistence of the testicle. There were symptoms of intestinal obstruction, but as the hernia was soft and compressible, with a gurgle, no operation was undertaken, and the patient died. On opening the abdomen no obstruction was at first found, but on closer examination a small 'buttonhole' was found in the 'iliac fossa,' and in this a small portion of the gut had been nipped, and was almost gangrenous. The testicle was found in connection with the sac of this hernia as a small atrophied particle. What was taken to be the testicle was a mass of fat, dense and hard.

This case is certainly not one of retro-colic hernia, but is a good example of how a case should not be recorded. No mention is made of the side, left or right, of the strangled segment of gut. We can but infer from the context that the left side is meant. If so, it is more than difficult to understand Jonnesco's reasons for including the case in his list of retro-colic herniæ.

The case bears, apparently, a fairly close resemblance to that of Fages already described.

Case of Furst.—A tailor, aged sixty-one. The body was examined in the dissecting-room. A very accurate and detailed report is given.

On opening the abdomen the cæcum was found to be below the umbilicus. The right hypochondriac and lumbar and a portion of the umbilical regions were occupied by a large peritoneal sac, the orifice of which measured in its largest diameter 12 centimetres, and looked downwards and a little forward and to the right. About two-thirds of the small intestine lay in the sac, the entering limb being the first part of the jejunum immediately beyond the flexura duodeno-jejunalis. The cæcum and ascending colon were on the inner wall of the sac, the rest of the large intestine being pushed well over to the left.

I do not propose to discuss this case fully. Many diverse opinions have been expressed about it. Furst considered that the sac was the result of an abnormal process occurring during the development of the peritoneum. Jonnesco attempts a similar explanation, but is in ignorance of the views of Toldt as to the fusion process in the normal peritoneal evolution. Brösike, regretting the lack of a detailed description of the duodenum and jejunum, concludes that the first part of the jejunum was adherent in a manner similar to that found by him when the recessus para-jejunalis is present. His argument attempts to show that the hernia has occurred into this fossa and has developed, in the irregular manner figured by Furst, on account of two reasons, firstly a free common mesentery for the cæcum and ascending colon, and secondly an unusually extended 'wandering' of the orifice of the mouth of the sac. This explanation appears to me to be very unlikely; but the case must be left at present undecided.

The only cases, then, that can, with any show of probability, be accepted as belonging to the class of retro-colic hernia are the last two of Rieux. All the others are negatived either by paucity and inexactness of description, or belong quite obviously to a different variety altogether.

This form of hernia, then, is very rare—rarer, in fact, than ileo-appendicular hernia.

RETRO-PERITONEAL HERNIA OF THE VERMIFORM PROCESS.

The above description excludes designedly any mention of hernia of the vermiform appendix. This small process is not infrequently found, on post-mortem examination, to be lying in the retro-colic fossa, or, more rarely, in the fossa of Hartmann, or in the ileo-appendicular fossa.

The subject has been studied closely by Lockwood alone among surgical writers. It is, however, of great importance, and deserves further and more extended investigation.

Lockwood, in his short article in the 'Transactions' of the Pathological Society, says that retro-peritoneal hernia of the vermiform appendix may occur into either the subcæcal (retrocolic) or ileo-cæcal (ileo-appendicular) fossæ; it may be partial or complete; the mouth of the fossa may be completely closed. Under this latter circumstance it may be exceedingly difficult to ascertain even the existence of the appendix. In one case that I have met with, a patient and careful search of the cæcum and its neighbourhood revealed no trace of the vermiform process. Any—even more than usually careful—observer might readily have been justified in concluding that the appendix was absent. I persisted in my search, however, and was rewarded eventually by finding a stunted process lying in a sac behind and rather to the inner side of the cæcum. The mouth of the sac was completely closed, and so smoothly and evenly that it was impossible to ascertain its existence without dissection. In the cases recorded as absence of the appendix, I cannot but think, with Lockwood, that some such condition as this has existed. One could only assert the absence of the process after a careful and complete dissection of the region.

Treves describes various positions of the vermiform appendix. That which he considers normal is one where the appendix points upwards and to the left towards the spleen. Between this position and one vertically behind the colon any direction may be assumed. Mettenheimer asserts that the normal position of the vermiform appendix is behind the cæcum and colon, whereas Turner of Moscow finds that its position is as follows: In 83 cases examined it was found in 51 to be in the true pelvis, and in 20 running transversely towards the sacral promontory. Bryant, of New York, gives a tabulated statement, showing that the four most common positions are 'inward,' 'downward and inward,' 'behind the cæcum,' and 'into the true pelvis.'

This exemplifies how diverse the opinions of various observers are—so diverse, indeed, as to be quite irreconcilable. I believe that this diversity is mainly due to an insufficiently extended observation. For in the first 100 cases that I observed, and of which I made note, in no fewer than

61 was the appendix hanging down in the true pelvis. In my second 100 I found that this position only occurred twenty-seven times, the most frequent in this series being the position which Treves considers normal. Taking the two series together, the pelvic position is a little more frequent than any other, but I hope to continue my observations for a much longer period, with the probability of arriving at a closer approximation to the average condition.

Lockwood and Rolleston describe the two positions (*a*) pointing to the spleen, and (*b*) hanging down into the pelvis, as the most usual for the vermiform appendix; and with 'a freely movable appendix it appears a matter of chance which of them is found. The appendix is easily displaced from one position to the other—so much so that we have hardly thought it possible to put it into correct statistical form.' I have, however, stated earlier on that I consider it not unlikely that the high or low position of the appendix may be in some definite relationship with the extent of the process of physiological adhesion that has occurred on the posterior surface of the ascending colon. At any rate, the point is worthy of further inquiry.

I do not propose to make any definite statement upon the frequency of retro-peritoneal hernia of the vermiform appendix, but I may mention that, speaking roughly, the condition may be said to exist in at least 8 or 10 per cent. of all subjects. That, I think, is rather under-estimating its frequency; but for the present it may be held to be approximately correct.

The importance of these positions in determining or influencing the occurrence of appendicitis can hardly be exaggerated.

HERNIA INTO THE FOSSA OF BIESIADECKI.

One example of this variety was exhibited at the London Pathological Society by Dr. Mott, who gives the following account: 'The vermiform appendix measured 7 inches. It turned up behind the cæcum, forming a sigmoid band, and terminated in a peculiar pouch $1\frac{1}{2}$ inches long in the anterior part of the iliac fossa. This pouch has been described as the infra- or retro-cæcal fossa. Mr. Treves termed it the fossa iliaco-subfascialis. There was apparently a small artery running along the pouch.'

The only other case that I have been able to find is that recorded by Engel, an epitome of which is given above. On the whole, I incline to agree with Leichtenstern, who considers the hernia to have been an example of this variety.

CHAPTER IV.

THE INTERSIGMOID FOSSA.

HISTORY.

The first mention of this fossa is made by Hensing, in the year 1742, in his Giessener dissertation already referred to: 'Antequam vero mesenterium relinquamus foramen quoddam cæcum mesenterii, notatu dignum non prætereundem est; nempe arca finem mesocoli sinistræ partis, ad latus sinistrum corporis primæ vertebræ ossis sacri, *semper atque constanter* foramen aliquid observavi, quod nullum exitum habet, atque valde, et ratione suæ circumferentiæ et profunditatis, in subjectis differt. Sæpissime enim circulus in de scripto loco solummodo adest, qui impressione aliqua levi, foramen quoddam repræsentat; interdum etiam foramen observatur, quod canalem versus centrum mesenterii tendentem et longitudinem trium unciarum habentem format; in eodem foramine interdum duo canales observantur; quorum unus versus centrum mesenterii, alter vero versus inferiora ossis sacri dirigitur.'

Roser in 1843 speaks of having seen the fossa very clearly defined on two occasions. In 1857 Engel speaks of a canal having a length of 3 centimetres in infants, extending along the inner border of the left psoas muscle to the level of the bifurcation of the aorta, and in exceptional cases as far up as the pancreas. He asserts that the fossa disappears in adults.

The best description is again given by Treitz, who says: 'Not infrequently there can be found in the mesocolon of the sigmoid flexure a depression or pocket of variable form and size. As a rule the fossa is about the size of a walnut or a hen's egg, reaching only seldom a length of 10 centimetres. Its upper closed end lies between the layers of the descending colon, while the opening is directed downwards. The margin of the opening is soft and smooth, so that in some cases, and especially in children, there may be merely a shallow depression. In the majority of cases, however, the edges of the opening are sharp, half-moon shaped, and may narrow or close the opening. These folds are the more frequently and the more plainly to be seen the younger the subject is.'

In 1859 Gruber applied the name 'retro-eversio hypogastrica sinistra seu inferior sinistra' to the fossa.

Waldeyer in his article already referred to describes the fossa and its more frequent varieties. He makes mention of a simple fossa, of two fossæ with a single opening, and of two fossæ opening by separate orifices.

In his Hunterian Lectures Treves has the following account: 'The pouch is formed between the layers of the mesocolon, and is due to a turning in of a funnel-shaped process of the peritoneum. The long axis of the pouch is directed downwards and to the left. The orifice is round or oval, with a distinct sharp edge that shows an absence of bloodvessels. The sigmoid artery lies above it and to the right. It is by the last-named vessel that the fossa is produced. The true fossa is not met with in small fœtuses. It is quite rare in the fœtus at full term, although at that period it is very often represented by a funnel-shaped depression. The perfect fossa was met with in 52 per cent. of all the subjects. But if distinct funnel-shaped depressions be added to the examples of the true fossa, then the percentage reaches 65.'

In 1890 Jonnesco gave a fairly accurate description of the fossa, describing two types, an 'infantile' and an 'adult.' He gives a most complicated, and to me utterly unintelligible, account of the genesis of the fossa. To this point I shall subsequently refer.

In 1892 Brösike gave an accurate account in his small work.

The genesis of the fossa has been dealt with accurately by Toldt and by Johnson Symington in 1892.

8

DESCRIPTION OF THE FOSSA.

On drawing the sigmoid or omega loop upwards and to the left, the left or under layer of the sigmoid mesocolon is exposed. On this surface can be seen the entrance to the intersigmoid fossa, at the line of insertion of the mesocolon (Fig. 32). The fossa is present in the greater number of bodies examined. Its frequency has been estimated at 60 per cent. by Gruber, 52 per cent. by Treves, 84 per cent. by Waldeyer, 70 per cent. by Jonnesco, and 53 per cent. by Eccles. My own experience shows that the fossa is present

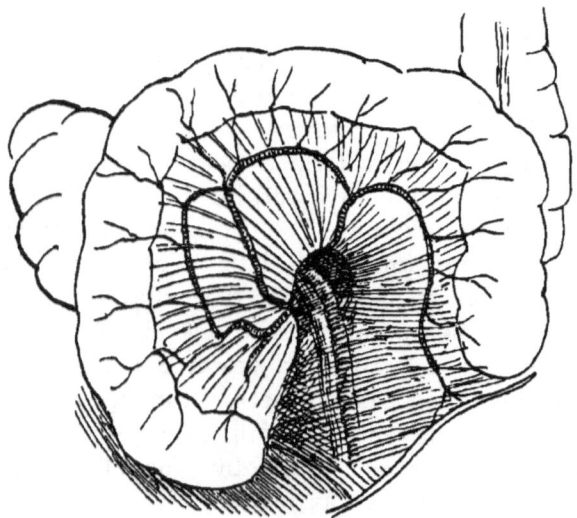

FIG. 32.—THE INTERSIGMOID FOSSA.

in a little over 70 per cent. of bodies examined. Its frequency depends, however, chiefly upon the ages of the subjects examined. In the fœtus of later months and in infants it is invariable. Its frequency becomes less with increasing years. As Treitz showed many years ago, in the aged there are never lacking signs of adhesion, crimping and thickening in the sigmoid mesocolon. Processes of this kind tend to obliterate all traces of the fossa, so that in subjects over fifty years of age the fossa is not infrequently wanting.

The opening of the pouch is situated in the line of attachment of the sigmoid mesocolon at a point which is near the inner margin of the psoas magnus. It lies over the common iliac artery, close to or in front of its bifurcation. The orifice is generally round or oval, and is bounded in front by a fairly well-defined sharp edge of peritoneum. In this peritoneal edge, or very close to it, may be found the sigmoid vessels. Behind the orifice is the parietal peritoneum, which, according to Engel, Gruber, and Waldeyer, may be raised up in the form of a sharp, stiff peritoneal fold, narrowing the opening.

This orifice leads to the intersigmoid fossa, which lies behind the sigmoid mesocolon and in front of the parietal peritoneum. The fossa has been frequently described as lying between the layers of the mesocolon (Treitz and Waldeyer), and Treves, for example, says: 'In other and less common instances the fossa is removed from the root of the mesocolon, and is found some way up upon that membrane—it may be midway between the parietes and the gut —or found even nearer to the bowel than to the attachment of the serous fold.' This statement is, I think, an exaggerated one. The fossa may certainly be found a little distance away from the parietal attachment of the mesocolon, but never, so far as my experience goes, as far up the fold as mentioned by Treves. Treves, moreover, does not say under what conditions this migration of the fossa occurs. It is only, I believe, in the aged that such a condition is found. Then, owing to distension and dragging of the sigmoid, due very possibly to constipation, the parietal peritoneum may be pulled upon, and with it the pouch, so that the orifice leaves the posterior wall entirely. In all cases, however, the distance between the gut and the fossa is that of the normal unaltered meso-sigmoid. The original position of the pouch, then, is behind the sigmoid mesocolon and in front of the parietal peritoneum.

The posterior wall of the fossa is adherent to the common iliac artery, and through the transparent wall can be seen the ureter as it crosses the vessel. The apex of the fossa extends upwards for a distance that varies very considerably.

Sometimes there is merely a dimple representing the fossa; in other cases the depth may be 2 or 3 inches, or even more. I have on several occasions seen the fossa extend beyond the middle of the kidney, and this is usually the case in fœtuses. Engel, Brösike, and Rogie describe the pouch as extending as far up as the body of the pancreas, and as we shall see in discussing the genesis of the fossa, this is not at all improbable. Most frequently the fossa is of the shape and size of an abbreviated glove-finger for an average middle finger.

Deviations from this normal state are occasionally seen, and have been described by the earlier authors. Hensing and Gruber speak of a fossa having a single orifice and two branches and of two separate fossæ.

Brösike has seen four fossæ closely placed together in a man thirty years of age. The significance of these variations will be referred to subsequently.

GENESIS OF THE FOSSA.

Several explanations have been suggested. The first is that of Treitz. To the views of this author I have already referred when speaking of the subcæcal fossæ. Treitz believed that the formation of the fossa was dependent upon and caused by the descent of the left testicle, just as the subcæcal fossa was dependent upon the descent of the right testicle. The fold described by him as the 'plica genito-enterica' pulled upon the descending mesocolon in such manner as to raise up a peritoneal fold bounding a pouch, the intersigmoid fossa.

Waldeyer attributed the formation of the pouch to the continued growth of the sigmoid mesocolon. 'During the increase of the sigmoid its mesentery tends to become elongated, and dragged more and more from the posterior abdominal wall. Thereby two vascular folds are raised up just in front of the ureter, and a pouch, funnel-shaped, comes to lie between them.'

Treves says briefly of the fossa that it is caused by the sigmoid artery.

Jonnesco gives a description of the origin of the fossa in language which to me is utterly and completely unintelligible. But whatever it may mean, the explanation which he attempts to give is wrong, and is written in ignorance or inappreciation of the work of Toldt in 1879. The account given by this author I have previously referred to.

In the early months of intra-uterine life the descending colon has a long mesentery attached near the middle line of the body. At about the sixth and seventh months the descending mesocolon is absent, and the descending colon lies in its adult position outside the kidney. This disappearance of the descending mesocolon was explained by Treitz, Luschka, Hyrtl, Waldeyer, and other observers as being due to the growth of the abdominal wall and the 'using up' of the mesocolon to form posterior parietal peritoneum. The layers of the serous fold were separated, it was said. The inaccuracy of these theories was first clearly shown by Toldt. He demonstrated that the disappearance of the mesentery of the descending colon was due to a process of 'physiological adhesion' taking place between the left (or posterior) layer of the mesocolon and the parietal peritoneum (Fig. 33). This agglutination begins above, close to the splenic flexure, and spreads gradually downwards. Over the kidney, owing to the projection of this organ, the fusion is earlier and more complete. Along the inner edge of the kidney is a groove, and here, therefore, the opposing surfaces do not so readily come into contact, and adhesion may be delayed. At the lower part of the groove union is never complete, and the gap that results is the intersigmoid fossa. The fossa thus formed lies along the inner margin of the kidney over the ureter, and opens below at the back of the sigmoid mesentery.

The process of physiological adhesion is generally completed by the seventh month. On examining a fœtus of this age, or a little younger, the descending mesocolon is obliterated. On pulling even gently on the colon, however, it will be found to strip up quite readily from the parietal peritoneum until the primitive mesocolon is reproduced. In doing this fine strands of connective tissue will be torn through. The process of agglutination has not been finally completed; the opposing surfaces are only loosely adherent. If a fine probe or bristle be previously passed into the intersigmoid fossa, this stripping up of the descending colon will lay it bare, lying behind the mesocolon and in front of the

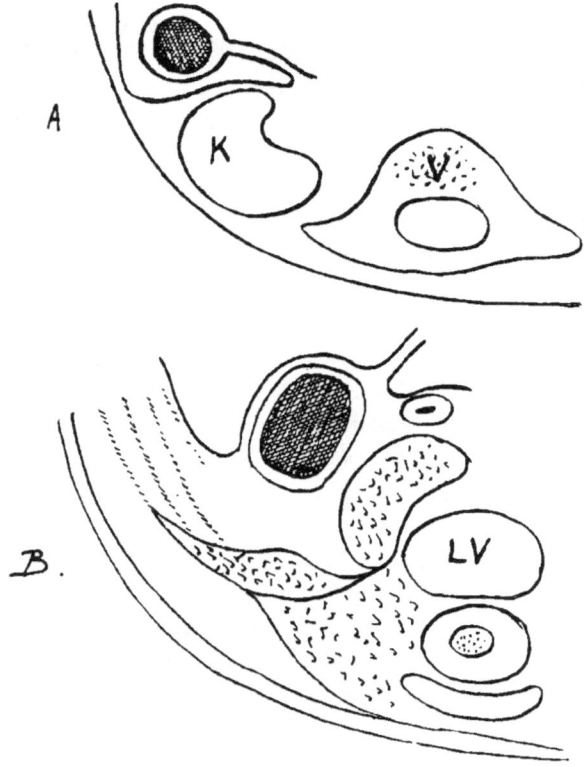

FIG. 33.—FORMATION OF THE INTERSIGMOID FOSSA.

A, Shows the descending mesocolon before the process of fusion has commenced; B, the descending mesocolon has disappeared, leaving the intersigmoid fossa on the inner side.

parietal peritoneum. This little experiment, which can be carried out, so far as I have seen, upon every fœtus of the latter end of the sixth or the beginning of the seventh month, proves conclusively the truth of Toldt's description.

This process of physiological agglutination will account also for the irregularities and abnormalities that are observed in the fossa. If the adhesion has been irregular, one, two, or more branches, or separate fossae, will be left, as in the cases previously referred to. The fusion, so far as I am aware, is never so complete as to obliterate the fossa altogether.

HERNIA INTO THE INTERSIGMOID FOSSA.

Treitz refers to two cases of intersigmoid hernia, one recorded by De Haen, and the other by Lawrence. De Haen describes and gives two figures of his case. Both the description and the figures negative decidedly the belief that the hernia was of the intersigmoid variety. It is a case of internal strangulation, and that is all that can be said of it. To some extent it resembles Jomini's case, to be quoted presently. Lawrence, in the fifth edition of his work, says that hernia may occur in the mesentery of the sigmoid, but gives no reference to a specific case.

The first case which has been definitely accepted by authors as one of intersigmoid hernia is recorded by Jomini. His description is as follows: Male, sixty-five years of age; dead on arrival at hospital. ' The abdominal tumour above mentioned is formed by a membranous sac, stretched and irregular on the surface, which is no other than the serous surface, unusually vascular by reason of the large vessels in it. This sac, covered by the omentum, is situate on the left at the level of the sigmoid flexure, and contains all the small intestine, with the exception of the upper third of the duodenum and the last centimetres of the ileum; the large intestine encircles it. This membranous pouch opens to the left of the vertebral column, on a level with the last lumbar vertebra, behind and below by an oval orifice with thick and fibrous edges. The orifice measures over 8 centimetres in its largest diameter, and allows the fist to enter easily. It is distant 7 to 9 centimetres from the descending colon and the sigmoid flexure. On its internal aspect the pouch is smooth, unaltered, covered by a membrane which is continuous with, and is part of, the general peritoneum. It corresponds to the peritoneal depression, which is found normally between the two leaves of the mesentery of the sigmoid, opening on the inferior. It receives the vessels of the left colic artery, one vessel almost encircling the orifice. On lifting the whole tumour up, some intestinal loops escape easily.' It is also stated that 'the duodenum contains biliary matters. At a few centimetres below the ampulla of Vater it enters the abdominal tumour.'

It is difficult to understand exactly what is meant by this inadequate description, which very unfortunately is unaccompanied by any figure. There is an obvious discrepancy in the two accounts given of the portion of duodenum entering the sac. At first it states that only 'the upper third' is outside the sac, and later that 'a few centimetres below the ampulla of Vater' it enters the abdominal tumour. Whichever description be accepted as correct, it is difficult to understand how the middle or lower portion of the duodenum could get on the left or under the surface of the sigmoid flexure unless it passed *behind* the mesocolon. And if it did so, what becomes of the enteric mesentery? and where was the duodeno-jejunal flexure? Brösike has discussed this case very critically, and decided that 'nie und nimmer' can it be accepted as one of intersigmoid hernia. To me, also, it seems quite impossible that it should be so. The case is very probably one of gross congenital abnormality of the original position of the whole intestinal canal. Later 'adhesion processes' have fixed the gut in its subsequent quite irregular position.

In June, 1885, Mr. F. S. Eve recorded the first authentic case of intersigmoid hernia. The specimen is now in the Museum of St. Bartholomew's Hospital (Fig. 34). I quote Mr. Eve's description: '*Necropsy.*—On opening the abdomen, I found the following condition: The intestines were injected and distended with flatus, but there was no effusion of lymph. On moving them aside to the right, it was observed that the sigmoid flexure was displaced towards the middle line, and extending from its posterior surface towards the left iliac fossa was a sheet of peritoneum, through an opening in which a knuckle of small intestine passed. The protruded intestine was withdrawn without the least resistance, and proved to be a portion, about 6 inches in length, of the lower end of the ileum. It was moderately congested, and was marked at each end by a slight constriction.

'The opening in the peritoneum (see Fig. 34 ƒ) was oval, and its long diameter measured ½ inch. It was situated close to the left side of the sigmoid flexure, its lower margin being from 1 inch to 1½ inches above and to the outer side of the sacro-iliac synchondrosis, and 1 inch from the ovary. On dissecting up the peritoneum from the subjacent muscles,

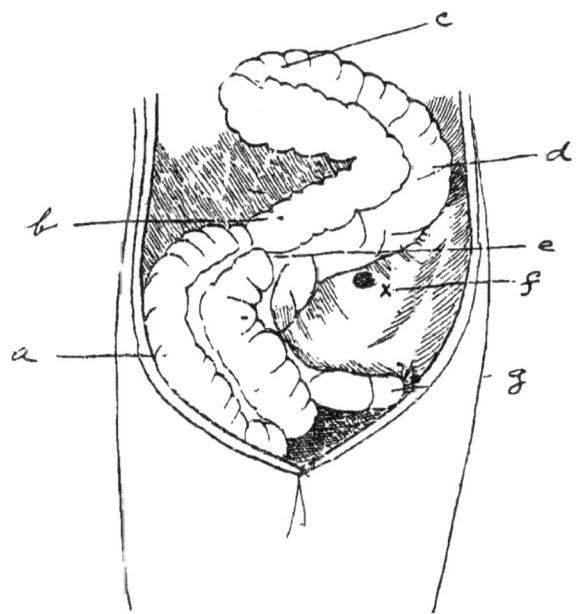

FIG. 34.—MR. EVE'S CASE OF INTERSIGMOID HERNIA.

the opening was found to lead into a sac of peritoneum having very thin walls, which were attached to or continuous with, the margins of the opening. The sac was pyriform, measured 3 inches in its long diameter, and extended upwards and backwards beneath the large intestine. Its posterior surface, in contact with the iliacus and lumbar muscles, was easily dissected from its connections; but its anterior surface was so closely connected with the peritoneum and posterior surface of the large bowel that its continuity in parts could not be established.

'The sigmoid flexure was nearly surrounded by peritoneum, but had not a distinct mesentery, the two layers of peritoneum reflected from it being nowhere in contact. Above the opening of the hernia the flexure was bound down to the iliac fossa by three bands of thickened peritoneum. The much-distended cæcum (*a*) occupied a position immediately to the right of the middle line.

'The ascending colon (*b*) took a course obliquely across the abdomen to the left hypochondrium, where it turned sharply to the right, and followed the curve of the diaphragm until it reached the middle line; here it became suddenly bent upon itself and returned, above and parallel to its previous course (*c*), to the lower edge of the spleen; thence it took the normal direction to the sigmoid flexure. Both the ascending and descending portions of the large intestine were closely united, and almost surrounded, by a single layer of peritoneum. A transverse colon, it need scarcely be said, did not exist.

'Just above the cæcum, the ascending colon and adjacent curve of the sigmoid flexure were bound together by a ribbon-like band of fibrous tissue (*e*) $\frac{3}{4}$ inch in breadth and $\frac{1}{2}$ inch in length; the adhesion to the flexure was 2 inches below the level of the hernial opening. The ascending colon was slightly narrowed by the tension to which the band gave rise, but the calibre of the lower bowel was unaltered, and, with the other large intestine, was of the usual dimensions.

'The upper end of the misplaced colon was connected by the great omentum to the great curvature of the stomach. In front of the sharp bend of the ascending colon at the middle line was a funnel-shaped pocket or cul-de-sac, 3 inches in length, which was formed by a depression or involution of peritoneum between the parallel running folds of large intestine.

'Part of the jejunum occupied the usual position of the ascending colon, and at a point 2 feet below the pyloric orifice had been opened and attached to the wound in the right loin, at which it presented during the operation.

'The condition of the large intestine offers some points of developmental and anatomical interest, which centre about the band of adhesion between the ascending colon and the sigmoid flexure. Presuming, as its appearance justifies, that this band was an adhesion formed at an early stage of development, the peculiar position of the large intestine becomes readily intelligible. The commencement of the ascending colon being tied to the lower part of the large bowel—which throughout development nearly retains its original position—the cæcum would be prevented from taking its usual course from the left hypochondrium to the right, and thence down to the right iliac fossa. Instead, it appears to have taken a direct path from the left hypochondrium obliquely across the abdomen to the right iliac fossa, carrying after it the ascending colon, which thus remains in close contact with the descending colon. The band appears likewise to have induced conditions favourable to the occurrence of hernia into the fossa intersigmoidea in the following manner. The left layer of the meso-sigmoidea being put upon the stretch by the displacement of the flexure towards the middle line, the orifice of the fossa would be rendered firm and immovable, and, further, may have been enlarged by the tension on the peritoneum around it. The importance of these collateral conditions is rendered forcibly apparent when the paucity of cases of intersigmoid hernia is contrasted with the constancy and occasionally large size of the fossa.

'The patient was a female, aged sixty-three, upon whom right lumbar "colotomy" was performed for intestinal obstruction.'

The most likely explanation of the history of this case is this: There had been originally a common mesentery for the jejunum, ileum, cæcum, and ascending colon. The splenic flexure and the descending colon became fixed in the usual manner by the adhesion of the left or posterior layer of the original descending mesocolon to the parietal peritoneum of the posterior abdominal wall.

As a result of peritoneal adhesion, most probably pathological, the cæcum and ascending colon had adhered to the descending colon and the sigmoid, and the united gut had been dragged over to the right, laying bare and rendering patent the orifice of the intersigmoid fossa.

A second case of intersigmoid hernia has been recorded by Mr. McAdam Eccles, who kindly sent me an account of his case, from which I abstract the following:

'A man, aged fifty-three, was admitted into the West London Hospital under my care on August 18, 1895, suffering from well-marked symptoms of intestinal obstruction. He gave the following history of his illness: For many years he had suffered from double inguinal hernia, for which he had worn a truss, and the instrument at most times answered its purpose satisfactorily. Both herniæ were easily reducible. On August 14, four days before admission, whilst he was coughing, the left rupture came down, and he found he was unable to reduce it. He says it felt very hard, and was very tender and painful. Soon after its protrusion he began to vomit, and nothing passed per anum; the pain also increased in severity at the seat of the hernia, and spread to the abdomen.

'He was soon after taken to the cottage hospital near where he lived, and admitted. He was seen by the surgeon with very little delay, and after some considerable difficulty the hernia was reduced by taxis.

'The vomiting and the pain, however, still persisted, and his bowels were only slightly opened by an enema, neither fæces nor flatus passing naturally.

'The pain did not subside, and the vomiting, which at first only came on after attempts to take food, occurred much more frequently.

'All the symptoms continued up to the time of his admission into the West London Hospital.

'He then exhibited the following symptoms: His face wore an anxious expression, and was also in other ways typical of acute abdominal disturbance. The pulse was small and frequent. His breathing was markedly thoracic, the tongue rather dry and thickly furred. Temperature, 98·2° F. The abdomen was full, being evenly distended, and everywhere resistant. No local swelling or induration could be made out. A resonant note could be elicited over the whole surface.

'Both inguinal regions were empty; no thickening of any

kind could be made out. But on invaginating the scrotum both external rings were found to be much enlarged, and the inguinal canals could be easily entered, and were discovered to be empty. There was no swelling in either femoral region. The patient vomited after admission, and the ejected matters had a distinctly fæculent odour. The urine was normal.

'Seeing that there were evident symptoms of intestinal obstruction, and that nothing could be palpated in the hernial regions, I decided to explore the abdominal cavity by a median laparotomy, rather expecting to find the results of a reduction *en masse*.

'After the patient had been placed under the influence of ether, an incision in the middle line was made of some 4 inches in length below the umbilicus. The abdominal wall was fairly well nourished and rather hyper-vascular. On opening the peritoneal cavity, blood-stained odourless fluid escaped. The left iliac fossa was explored. The left internal abdominal ring was not occupied by any protrusion, and admitted the finger.

'Lying, however, rather higher up in the fossa, and at the posterior part of the abdomen, was a firm resistant mass, into which could be traced small intestine, one part of which was distended and the other collapsed.

'It was plain that this constituted the seat of obstruction.

'A closer examination revealed a tightly-constricting edge, which afterwards proved to be the margin of the aperture of the intersigmoid fossa.

'The tight sharp ring was carefully snipped with a pair of scissors, and the gut slowly drawn out of its grasp.

'A loop of small intestine was thus liberated, which was intensely congested, with a length of about half an inch in its middle black and gangrenous.

'The whole loop measured about 4 inches, and it was brought out of the abdominal wound.

'Two pieces of rubber drainage-tube of small calibre were passed through the mesentery, close to the intestine, at points which were some 3 inches beyond the congested part on either side.

'The gangrenous piece of bowel, with the œdematous portion, was entirely excised, together with a V-shaped piece of mesentery. The contents of the upper dilated portion of small intestine were allowed to freely escape through the open end, and when fairly empty the rubber tube was drawn tight and secured at both places.

'The extremities of the healthy bowel were now united by Maunsell's method.

'The loop being washed and returned, the peritoneal cavity was sponged out and the abdominal wound closed.

'The patient stood the operation, which lasted fifty minutes, very fairly well, and rallied afterwards.

'The vomiting and pain, however, recurred some six hours after the patient returned to the ward, and he died of exhaustion about twelve hours later.

'The post-mortem examination showed some general peritonitis, most marked in the region of the sigmoid flexure, which was itself thrown over to the right side of the body. There were no evidences of old peritonitis in the form of adhesions, all the inflammation present being of a recent nature. The sutures used in the anastomosis had held well, and there was but little distension of the gut above the resected portion.'

This is an exceedingly interesting case, for it shows that intersigmoid hernia may occur in a normal peritoneal cavity. There were no signs of any old peritonitis; there was no abnormality in size or position of the sigmoid flexure or any part of the large intestine.

The only two cases of intersigmoid hernia that we can accept, then, are Mr. Eve's and Mr. Eccles'. And they illustrate as well as possible two quite opposite conditions. In the one there was congenital abnormality, gross in extent, and peritoneal adhesion probably pathological and extrauterine, and in the other a peritoneal cavity in all respects normal.

CHAPTER V.

THE FORAMEN OF WINSLOW.

ANATOMY.

THE foramen of Winslow is the aperture of communication between the greater and lesser sacs of peritoneum. It is bounded above by the caudate lobe of the liver, below by the duodenum and the hepatic vessels; in front by the lesser omentum, containing the hepatic artery, portal vein and bile-duct, and behind by the vena cava. In size it is variable, but will as a rule admit one finger easily. In the earlier years of life the foramen, which looks forwards and to the right, is clearly defined, and seen quite distinctly by dragging the liver upwards. In later years it is not unusual to find a certain number of adhesions between the anterior and posterior boundaries of the orifice. In some cases, as a result of gall-stone irritation, the adhesions are very firm and tough, and completely obliterate the entrance to the lesser sac. In many of Mr. Mayo Robson's operations for gall-stones in the gall-bladder, cystic, or common ducts, I have seen the adhesions so numerous and so firm as to render it a matter of impossibility to recognise the normal anatomical landmarks. This point, indeed, was referred to by Treitz many years ago, but its significance was not appreciated.

HERNIA INTO THE FORAMEN OF WINSLOW.

This form of hernia is very uncommon. I have been able to find only 8 cases recorded, 4 very imperfectly by Rokitansky, Treitz, Moir, and Novello, and 4 more fully by Blandin, Majoli, Elliot-Square, and Treves. The reasons for the infrequency of its occurrence are not difficult to understand. As Engel long ago remarked, 'the transverse colon forms a strong natural barrier to the passage of the small intestine towards the foramen.' Moreover, the foramen is very probably potential rather than actual. Its anterior and posterior ligamentary boundaries are, as a rule, in contact with one another.

After reading carefully the reports of all the recorded cases, it seems to me almost certain that in order to permit of the occurrence of this form of hernia there must be some gross congenital abnormality. In the carefully-recorded cases this has been observed. Thus, in Treitz's case there was 'a common mesentery for the intestine from the duodenum to the rectum.' In the cases reported by Elliot-Square and Treves there was an absence of the secondary fusion process between the ascending colon and the posterior abdominal wall.

If the secondary adhesion is absent, and the ascending colon and the hepatic flexure have not undergone their usual migration to the right, then the foramen will be unduly large and patulous. Probably in Majoli's case there was some aberration from the normal. In the earlier cases no mention is made of any relevant observation. The records, however, are very paltry and insufficient. It is possible that an abnormally long mesentery, as in the cases described by Lockwood in his Hunterian Lectures, may be a predisposing cause also.

We may tabulate the causes, then, as:

1. A common mesentery for the whole intestine. Rogie (*Journ. des Sci. Méd. de Lille*, 1892) has collected 53 examples from the literature of the subject, and he has not included all the cases.

2. Absence of the secondary fusion of the ascending colon to the posterior abdominal wall.

3. Abnormally large size of the foramen of Winslow.

4. Abnormal length of the mesentery, and consequently undue mobility of the intestine.

In the absence of one or other of these abnormalities, the occurrence of the hernia may be considered almost a physical impossibility.

The following cases of hernia into the foramen of Winslow are recorded:

1. *Rokitansky.*—'I have on one occasion seen a large portion of the small intestine strangled by the foramen of Winslow.'

2. *Blandin* (also referred to by Jobert, *Traité Théorique et Pratique des Maladies Chirurgicale du Canal Intestinal,* 1829).—'The patient was admitted to the Charité suffering from acute peritonitis. At the autopsy a large segment of the small intestine entered the foramen of Winslow; a portion of this segment left the lesser cavity of the peritoneum by an opening in the transverse colon. At this opening the gut was strangled.'

3. *Treitz.*—A woman aged thirty-three. There was a common mesentery for the whole intestinal canal from the duodenum to the rectum. Two loops of the jejunum passed through the foramen of Winslow into the lesser sac. Treitz remarks: 'I have sometimes seen the large intestine, and especially the hepatic flexure of the colon or an abnormally increased loop of the transverse colon in the foramen of Winslow.'

4. *Dr. Wilson Moir, of Musselburgh* (quoted by Chiene).—A case observed in Vienna. The patient died with symptoms of internal strangulation. 'On opening the abdomen the small intestine was invisible; on closer inspection it was found to have passed into the lesser cavity of the peritoneum through the foramen of Winslow.'

5. *Majoli* (this account is copied from Treves' article subsequently referred to).—An emaciated man, the subject during the greater part of his life of chronic constipation, presented a persistent bulging of the anterior abdominal wall in the epigastric region, somewhat more to the right than to the left. A painful, rounded tumour, dull on percussion, was readily defined in this situation. Symptoms of obstruction of the bowel were present. The diagnoses of fæcal accumulation or of colic intussusception were proposed. Enemata were employed, and doses of metallic mercury were given, but without effect. The man died fifteen days after the stone of the symptoms. The necropsy revealed a loop of

the transverse colon strangulated in the foramen of Winslow. The bowel was gangrenous.

6. *Alpago Novello* (referred to by Majoli).—A loop of small intestine 2 metres in length had passed through the foramen of Winslow.

7. *Elliot Square.*—' R. F., aged twenty-five, a clerk, was apparently in perfect health when he sat down to his dinner at noon on May 7. He made a good meal of beefsteak-pie and potatoes, and walked to his office as usual, a distance of about a quarter of a mile. Without any apparent cause whatever, about two o'clock he was suddenly seized with excruciating pain in the epigastrium. He walked home at once with difficulty, and was " doubled up with pain." He was given brandy-and-water and a dose of castor-oil, after which he vomited for the first time about four o'clock. Pain and vomiting continued, with sleepless nights, until the 9th, when he was so much easier that in the afternoon he sat out by the fire; but in the evening his symptoms returned as severe as ever.

'At seven o'clock on the evening of the 10th I saw him for the first time; practically nothing until then had been done for him. I found him in bed in a most excited state, his face anxious and somewhat pinched, his temperature 103·4° in the axilla, and his pulse 122, regular and small. His parents had had great difficulty in keeping him in bed, and had found it quite impossible to keep the bedclothes upon him. They were very inexperienced and foolishly nervous people, had none of his vomit to show me, and quite misinformed me as to its character; he had not vomited for an hour or two. The legs were not drawn up, and he said that he had then no pain, but that the pain over the ensiform cartilage, and immediately below it, had been excruciating. The abdomen looked natural, except that the umbilicus was somewhat prominent; in infancy he had worn an umbilical pad. Percussion and manipulation gave no pain, except around the umbilicus and in the epigastrium, where there was decided tenderness. The abdomen was everywhere resonant, except in the flanks—very resonant over the transverse colon. The bowels had not acted since the morning of the 6th; the urine contained no albumen.

'Feeling certain that there was an intestinal obstruction, I accordingly gave orders for treatment, and administered an injection of warm water and soap. Three hours afterwards I returned, and finding that there had been no relief, gave a second larger injection, which soon brought away what might be termed a diarrhœa stool, with two solid fæcal masses. This gave him great encouragement, and, after giving fresh instructions, and having arranged for an early consultation, I again left him.

'The vomit was now fæcal, though without the offensive smell. At 3 a.m., in answer to an urgent summons, I was again at his bedside. He was much changed, and was in the most childish condition; we could neither keep him in bed nor prevent him from throwing off the bedclothes; his restlessness was intense. His hands and feet were cold and clammy, and his pulse feeble, though he was quite conscious. He was given three small hypodermic injections of morphine at intervals of about two minutes, and I left him, moderately quiet, at 4.30. He became quieter, and sank at seven o'clock, after an illness of three days and seventeen hours.

'The examination of the body was obtained with the greatest difficulty, and was performed at great inconvenience, without skilled assistance. On opening the abdomen, a moderate amount of peritonitis was at first noticeable, with a small amount of lymph and bloody serum among the intestines. The umbilicus was quite free. The great omentum was drawn in among the small intestines, to the left of the middle line, and was moderately congested. The intestines contained only a very small quantity of fæcal matter, but were distended with gas. Fully 8 inches of the ileum, about 2 feet from its termination in the cæcum, were firmly incarcerated in the foramen of Winslow, and were with some difficulty withdrawn. Its mesentery was much congested; the intestine itself much more so; and though, at the junction of the two, there were three or four soft disintegrating patches, in no part was there found any perforation or ulceration through the coats of the intestine.

On withdrawing the intestine the foramen gaped, and would easily admit two fingers; its margins were rounded, thickened, and congested. The cæcum was freely movable, and possessed a mesocæcum. Had an operation been performed at an early date, I have every reason to believe it would have been successful.'

8. *Treves.*—The account of Mr. Treves' case is contained in a most admirable clinical lecture on 'Hernia into the Foramen of Winslow,' published in the *Lancet*, October 13, 1888:

'The patient was a good type of a well-developed, muscular, and robust man. He had "never had a day's illness in his life," was of steady habits, knew nothing of dyspepsia, and never suffered from constipation. He had certainly been free from any intestinal trouble previous to the attack which caused his death. On April 9 he ate a very hearty dinner at 3 p.m., concluding the meal with a considerable number of periwinkles. At 5 p.m. he was suddenly seized with violent abdominal pain. The pain was like cramp, and was situate about and above the umbilicus. He was bent double, became faint, and broke out into a cold perspiration. He drank some brandy, which was retained. The pain was intermittent, the intervals of freedom from pain, however, being very short. The abdomen was not tender. The pain persisted all night, and was of such a character that he could not lie down, but spent the night in a chair. Before the morning the abdomen began to be a little distended, and to feel "tight" in the epigastrium. On the 10th he began to vomit, rejecting some milk he had swallowed. The pain was still severe and intermittent, and was still in the same situation. Nothing had passed the rectum since the morning of the previous day. Dr. Ambrose found the abdomen everywhere tympanitic, the meteorism being especially marked in the epigastric region, where, and where only, the abdomen appeared a little swollen. An examination of the rectum and of the cæcal region revealed nothing. The patient was sick about ten times during the day. Opium was now administered in doses that represented about 3 grains of opium powder in twenty-four hours. On the next day (the 11th) the pain was much less severe; but the vomiting continued, the patient being sick from ten to fifteen times in the twenty-four hours. On the 12th the bowels were well relieved, for the first time since the onset, by an enema. The patient was much easier, and vomited only once during the day. The tongue was now coated. The abdomen was more evenly distended, and was tympanitic everywhere, although the percussion note varied greatly in degree in different parts. The distension in the regions below the umbilicus was much reduced by the injection, and the swelling in the epigastrium was thereby rendered more distinct. This swelling occupied more or less precisely the epigastric area as anatomically defined, and appeared to be due to the distended stomach and colon. On the following day no change was to be noted. The bowels again acted after an enema, the patient felt better, and was only sick twice. Nothing passed the rectum after this date, in spite of copious and repeated enemata. During the three succeeding days (the 14th, 15th, and 16th) the patient's troubles increased. The pain again became severe, but was no longer intermittent, although it presented variations in its intensity. Vomiting occurred from twelve to fifteen times in the twenty-four hours. The epigastric swelling was more distinct, and on the 16th was noticed to be a little dull on percussion for the first time. There was no localized abdominal tenderness. As evidence of the man's general condition, it is noted that on the 15th he insisted on leaving his bedroom for some hours, and walked downstairs without assistance. On April 17 the patient was admitted into Dr. Mackenzie's wards. Before describing his condition when he entered the hospital, I might mention some general facts in the history of the week that had intervened since the attack came on. The treatment had consisted in rest, in the frequent use of enemata, in fomentations to the abdomen, in a most restricted diet, and in the daily administration of 3 grains of opium. The pain had always been complained of as about and above the umbilicus. It had at first been intermittent, but later had exhibited only variations in intensity. It had been of the character of cramp or colic.

No specific tenderness had ever been complained of. During the whole of the week the patient had kept the sitting posture, declaring that he was unable to lie down. The vomiting had been throughout slight in amount; it was at first purely gastric and ultimately intestinal. It was never feculent. The sickness gave the patient no relief, and except on two days (April 13 and 14) whatever was taken by the mouth was rejected, although not directly. There had never been hiccough. An almost constant tenesmus had marked the whole progress of the trouble. The urine was normal, was of high specific gravity, and moderate in amount. The tongue was at first clean, but soon became coated and flabby, and on April 15 dry and brown. The pulse throughout had been small and regular, and had varied from 85 to 100. The temperature had been normal or subnormal, and had averaged 98°. There had been almost complete loss of appetite, with great thirst. Dyspnœa had never been complained of. Intestinal movements were at no time visible, nor were borborygmi heard. The skin had been usually moist. The loss of strength had been gradual, and the patient's intelligence had remained clear. There had been no discharge from the rectum. When Dr. Mackenzie and I examined the patient, we found him in a condition of great prostration, with the pinched face and sunken eyes of acute abdominal trouble. The tongue was dry and brown, the temperature subnormal, the pulse 98, small and feeble. The patient was now lying upon the back, with the knees drawn up. Nothing had passed the rectum for three days. A little brownish fluid with a faint intestinal odour was being vomited about every half-hour. There was still much pain about the umbilicus. The abdomen was moderately distended, but there was a very conspicuous bulging of the anterior abdominal wall in the epigastric and hypochondriac regions. The summit of this swelling was in the median line. In the left hypochondriac district a high resonant note was elicited on percussion, and appeared to indicate a distended stomach. The whole of the area defined anatomically as the epigastric was dull, although a resonant note could be produced on deep percussion. Elsewhere the abdomen was evenly tympanitic. There was tenderness in the epigastrium, and it was evident that this region was the seat of some peritonitis. A rectal examination revealed nothing. The even swelling above the umbilicus rendered the aspect of the abdomen quite peculiar.

'Such are the clinical facts of the case. So far as diagnosis went, it was only possible to say with certainty that there was an obstruction involving the colon, that this obstruction was complete, and probably concerned the bowel not far from its commencement, and, moreover, that there was some peritonitis in the epigastric region. There was no evidence to support the diagnosis of intussusception, the symptoms did not accord with the conception of a mesenteric or mesocolic (retro-peritoneal) hernia, there was evidence that the case was not one of volvulus of the sigmoid flexure, and the nearest approach to probability appeared to lie in the suggestion of a volvulus of an undescended cæcum. In the light, however, of the present case, and the few other examples of hernia into the foramen of Winslow which have been recorded, I believe it possible that in future the lesion may possibly be diagnosed during life.

'As the patient's condition was very urgent, and as both he and his friends were most anxious that no possible effort to save his life should be spared, Dr. Mackenzie advised an exploratory incision, and in this advice I entirely concurred. The operation was performed on the afternoon of April 17, precisely eight days after the commencement of the attack. I opened the abdomen in the median line below the umbilicus, and introduced my hand. I first sought the cæcum, but neither it nor the ascending colon was to be found. I then passed to the left colon, and found that the descending colon, sigmoid flexure, and rectum were empty and flaccid. I endeavoured to follow the upper end of the descending colon, but found it impossible to do so owing to the distension of the adjacent coils of small intestine and the presence of a dilated stomach. I now turned my attention to the small intestine, and soon discovered that there was no true mesentery. I, however, followed a coil of the bowel until I reached a constricting ring in the epigastric region through which this bowel passed. At first it appeared probable that the ring might be the opening of the fossa duodeno-jejunalis, and the case one of retro-peritoneal hernia. The ring was, however, above the situation of that fossa, and had no direct relation to the vertebral column. Moreover, the sac of a mesenteric hernia could not be made out, while by following the aorta the true situation of the duodeno-jejunal fossa could be demonstrated. The orifice through which the coil of intestine passed was considerably to the right and above the usual situation of the mouth of the sac in mesocolic hernia. By a process of exclusion rather than by direct evidence it became clear that the constricting ring was the foramen of Winslow, but the presence of distended and unaccountable coils of intestine in the vicinity of the opening rendered the demonstration of the relations very difficult. The relation with the stomach could not be defined, and the presence of greatly dilated bowel served to confuse its position with reference to the liver. In the tissues in front of the ring an artery, clearly the hepatic, could be felt pulsating. I managed to reduce, with but little difficulty, some 2 or 3 feet of small intestine. The reduction, however, of another and quite distinct coil which also occupied the ring was utterly impossible. It was also impossible to enlarge the opening through which the bowel had passed, for even modern abdominal surgery has not proved that the hepatic artery, the portal vein, and the bile-duct can be divided simultaneously with impunity. Further attempts to relieve the patient had therefore to be abandoned. The patient never rallied after the exploratory operation, and died some six hours after he had been carried back to bed.

'The condition made evident at the necropsy is known to many of you. There was commencing general peritonitis. When the abdominal cavity was fully exposed, a coil of large intestine, so enormously distended as to be 4 inches in diameter, was found lying in the left hypochondriac region immediately under the costal cartilages of the left side. Below it the stomach, slightly distended and somewhat displaced forwards and to the left, presented itself. No other viscera were to be seen except the liver and coils of the small intestine. No other portion of the colon was in view (Fig. 35). Further examination showed that the cæcum, the whole of the ascending colon, and a part of the transverse colon had passed through the foramen of Winslow, and had become strangulated by the margin of that aperture. The colon, on entering the snare, had passed from right to left;

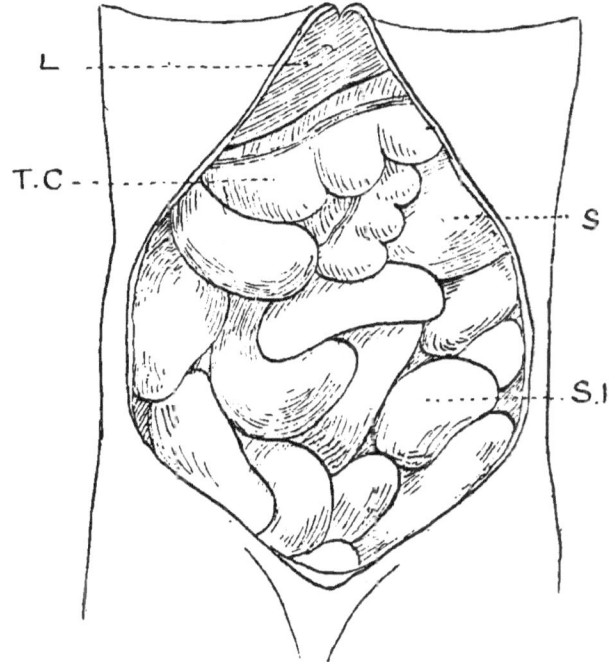

FIG. 35.—ASPECT OF PARTS ON OPENING THE ABDOMEN. (TREVES.)

the cæcum was to the extreme left of the abdominal cavity, and had forced its way through the anterior layer of the gastro-hepatic omentum, so that the vermiform appendix was actually lying on the anterior aspect of the lesser curvature of the stomach, close to the œsophagus (Fig. 36). The diameter of the strangulated colon measured nearly 5 inches. This part of the bowel was gangrenous in two places. Both patches were limited to the ascending colon; one patch was equal in size to a half-crown piece, while the other was twice as large. The intestine had given way a little in the latter situation, and fæcal matter had found its way into the lesser cavity of the peritoneum. The colon outside or beyond the foramen of Winslow turned very sharply to the left, and was then represented by the distended segment of the large intestine, already described as lying above the stomach (Fig. 37). On reaching the splenic flexure, the bowel was so sharply bent upon itself as to be again occluded. This kinking accounted for the great dilatation of that portion of the transverse colon which lay beyond the seat of strangulation. The descending colon, sigmoid flexure, and rectum were empty

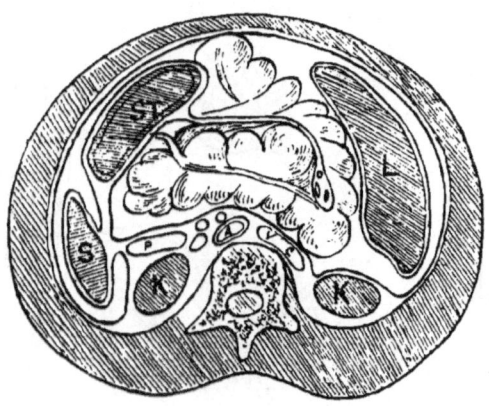

Fig. 36.—Section (diagrammatic) of the Abdomen at the Level of the Foramen of Winslow, showing the Hernia in situ. (Treves.)

and collapsed. The great omentum was found rolled up along the greater curvature of the stomach. The whole of the small intestine was distended. Some 4 or 5 inches of the terminal parts of the ileum were still found within the hernial cavity. It had passed in with the cæcum, but was only partially strangulated. The 2 or 3 feet of ileum that had been reduced during the operation were indicated by a purplish discoloration as compared with the rest of the intestine. At the seat of stricture the colon was in front of the small intestine. Of the strangulated colon the cæcum was the part that had suffered least. There was a descending mesocolon of moderate length. The colon may be described as being very sharply bent upon itself at the foramen of Winslow. The situation of this acute bending—the seat of the stricture—would correspond to about the centre of the transverse colon. The bowel from this point to the top of the cæcum was involved in the strangulation. The remaining (distal) half of the transverse colon was dilated by reason of the abrupt manner in which the bowel was again bent upon itself at the splenic flexure. This portion of the intestine (the distal half of the transverse colon) showed merely the effects of great distension. In other respects it was normal.

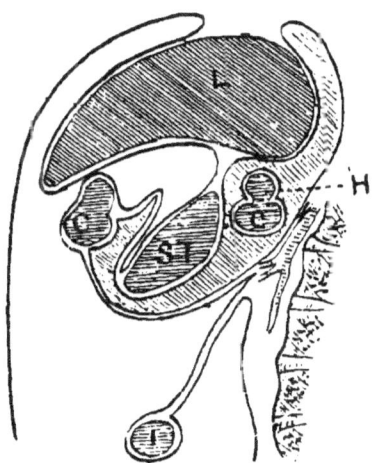

Fig. 37.—Vertical Section (diagrammatic) to show the Position of the Ascending and Transverse Portions of the Colon. (Treves.)

There was, of course, no trace of a hepatic flexure. There was a considerable degree of peritonitis in the epigastric area, and a few fresh adhesions united the ascending colon to the liver. The liver showed no morbid change of any kind. The stomach was merely distended. All the other viscera were perfectly normal. It was evident that the cæcum was "undescended," and had led the way through the foramen. The foramen of Winslow admitted four fingers. The tissues about it appeared normal, and no change could be detected in the structures occupying the gastro-hepatic omentum. The gall-bladder was but moderately full. It was found to be quite impossible to reduce the strangulated colon. Traction was maintained until the peritoneal coat of the bowel began to give way. Reduction could not be accomplished until the hepatic artery, the portal vein, and the bile-duct had been divided.'

SYMPTOMS.

On analyzing the series of cases, it seems that a hernia into the foramen of Winslow which becomes strangulated presents a fairly well-marked group of symptoms. These are:

1. *Pain.*—This is generally epigastric. Square speaks of 'pain over the ensiform cartilage and immediately below it.' Treves of 'pain like cramp at and above the umbilicus.' Majoli of 'a painful rounded tumour' in the epigastrium.

2. *Tumour.*—An epigastric tumour has generally been observed. Thus Majoli says 'a persistent bulging of the anterior abdominal wall in the epigastric region' was present.

Treves speaks of 'a conspicuous bulging of the anterior abdominal wall in the epigastric and hypochondriac regions.' Square says 'the umbilicus was somewhat prominent.'

3. *Percussion.*—A tumour, when present, is dull on light percussion, but deep percussion sounds a fairly resonant note.

In a typical case, then, we should expect to find:

Acute intestinal obstruction, with intense, almost intolerable epigastric pain, with epigastric prominence or tumour, such prominence being dull on superficial, slightly resonant on deep, percussion. It is interesting to note that there are no recorded symptoms of pressure on the hepatic artery, portal vein, or bile-duct.

TREATMENT.

So far as our present knowledge goes, the only possible treatment would be enterostomy, the formation of an artificial anus. In cases where the strangulation occurs at the foramen it has been found impossible to withdraw the congested gut from the lesser sac. Where the strangulation occurs through an opening out of the lesser bag, it is obvious that the condition could not be dealt with by withdrawal of the gut. The only course open to the surgeon is the formation of an artificial anus. Treves remarks of his case that the reduction of the hernia could only have been made possible by the simultaneous division of the hepatic artery, portal vein, and common bile-duct. Such a drastic measure as this is not yet to be counted as one of the achievements of modern surgery.

ALPHABETICAL LIST OF REFERENCES.

ALBERS. Atlas der pathologischen Anatomie. Mit Erläuterungen. IV. Abth.

ANDERSON, R. J. Notes on a Case of Abnormal Arrangement of the Peritoneum. Journal of Anatomy and Physiology, vol. xii., part ii., 1878.

BAGIGNI. Zwei neue Fälle von innerer Darmeinklemmung nebst einigen Bemerkungen über die Zweckmassigkeit der Enterotomie. Pistoja (Gaz. Toscana, 5, 1847).

BARBETTE. Chirurgia, pars i., cap. viii.

BARDELEBEN. Ueber die Lage des Blinddarms bein Menschen. Virchow's Archiv., 1849, Bd. II.

BARDENHEUER. Der extraperitoneale Explorativschnitt. Die differentielle Diagnostik der chir. Erkrankungen und Neubildungen des Abdomen. Stuttgart, 1887.

BARTH. Bull. de la Soc. Anat., Paris, 24ᵉ année, 1849, Bd. IV.

BESNIER. Des Étranglements internes de l'Intestin, etc. Mémoire couronnée par l'Académie de Médecine (Prix Portal de 1859). Paris, 1860.

BIESIADECKI. Fossa iliaco-subfascialis, Untersuchungen aus dem path. Anatom. Institut zu Krakau (s. bei Tarenetzki).

BLANDIN. Traité d'Anatomie topographique ou Anatomie du Corps humain, 2ᵉ édit., 1834.

BOCHDALEK, JUN. Ueber den Peritonealuberzug der Milz u. s. w. Archiv. für Anat., Physiol. und wissenschaftliche Medicin. Jahrg. 1867.

BORDENAVE. Mémoires de l'Académie royale des Sciences (MDCCLXXXII.), année 1779.

BREISKY. Casopis leraku ceskych, 1862. Med. Jahrbuch. Wien, 1863. Prag, 1857.

BARRS. A Case of Strangulated Retro-Peritoneal Hernia. Lancet, August, 1891.
BRUGNOLI. Quoted by Lambl. Vierteljahrschrift für die praktische Heilkunde. Sechszehnter Jahrgang, 1859. I. Band.
BERRY, R. J. A. The Cæcal Folds and Fossæ and the Topographical Anatomy of the Vermiform Appendix. Edinburgh, 1897.
BRYANT, J. D. Topographical Anatomy of the Vermiform Appendix. Annals of Surgery, February, 1893, p. 164.

CHIENE. Anatomical Description of a Case of Intra-Peritoneal Hernia. Journal of Anatomy and Physiology, 1868, vol. ii.
CRUVEILHIER. Bulletin de la Société Anatomique, 2ᵉ année, mai, 1827; et Traité d'Anatomie descriptive, tome ii., 5ᵉ édit., 1874-76.
CLARKE, J. JACKSON. A Case of Retro-Peritoneal Hernia. Pathological Society Transactions, vol. xliv., 1893, p. 67.
COOPER, ASTLEY. The Anatomy and Surgical Treatment of Crural and Umbilical Hernia, part ii. London, 1807.

DEVILLE. 1. Bull. de la Soc. Anat. Paris, 24ᵉ année, 1849.
2. Bull. de la Soc. Anat. Paris, 26ᵉ année, 1851.
DUCHAUSSOY. Anatomie pathologique des Étranglements internes et conséquences pratiques qui en découlent. Mémoire couronnée par l'Académie Impériale de Médecine (1859). Mémoire de l'Académie Impériale de Médecine, tome xxiv., 1860.

ENGEL. 1. Einige Bemerkungen über Lageverhältnisse der Baucheingeweide im gesunden Zustande. Wiener med. Wochenschrift, 1857.
2. Anatomische Mittheilungen für die Praxis. Wiener med. Wochenschrift, No. 36, September 7, 1861.
EPPINGER. Hernia Retro-Peritonealis. Vierteljahrschrift für die Pract. Heilkunde, 1870. Jahrg. xxvii., Bd. I., Prag.
EVE. A Case of Strangulated Hernia into the Fossa Intersigmoïde. British Medical Journal, June 13, 1885, No. 1276.
ECCLES, W. MCADAM. Case of Strangulation of a Loop of Small Intestine in the Fossa Intersigmoidea. St. Bartholomew's Hospital Reports, vol. xxxi., p. 177.

FAGES. Recueil Périodique de la Société de Médecine de Paris, tome vii., 1ᵉʳ Septembre de l'an VIII. de la République.

FAUCON. Sur une Variété de l'Étranglement interne, reconnaissant pour Causes les Hernies Internes ou Intra-Abdominales. Archives Générales de Médecine, 6 série, tome xxi., 1873.

FURST. Nordiskt Mediciniskt Arkiv., redigeradt af Axel Key. Sextonde Bandet, Tredje Häftet. Stockholm, 1884.

FOWLER, G. RYERSON. Observations upon Appendicitis. Annals of Surgery, vol. xix., 1894, pp. 4 *et seq.*

GRUBER.   1. Cit. Bericht. Med. Ztg. Russlands, 1859.
        2. Ueb. d. Hernia int. Mesogastrica. St. Petersburger Med. Ztg., 1861, Bd. I.
        3. Zur Hernia Interna. St. Petersburger Med. Ztg., 1862, Bd. II.
        4. Bildungshemmung d. Mesenterien. Archiv. für Anat. und Physiol., 1862 und 1864.
        5. Hernia int. Mesogastrica. Oesterr. Zeitschrift für Praktische Heilkunde, 1863, Wien.
        6. Nachträge z. d. Bildungshemm. d. Mesent., Hernia int. Mesogastr. Dextra. Virchow's Archiv., Bd. XLIV. Berlin, 1868.
        7. Fall von Mesent. Commune, etc. Virchow's Archiv., Bd. XLVII., 1869.

GONTIER. Hôpital Beaujon, service de M. Moutard-Martin. Union Médicale, III. série, tome viii., 1869.

GOSSELIN. Leçons sur les Hernies Abdominales, recueillies par Léon Labbé, 1865.

GÉRARD-MARCHANT. Quoted in Jonnesco's work, pp. 89-91, etc.

HALLER. Elementa Physiologiæ corp. hum., vol. vii.

HARTMANN. Die Bauchfelltaschen in der Umgebung des Blinddarms. Inaugural-Dissertation zur Erlangung der Doctorwürde. Tübingen, 1870.

HAUFF. Beiträge zur Pathol. Anatomie in Chr. Schmidt's Jahrbücher der in- und ausländischen gesammten Medicin. Jahrgang 1839, Bd. XXIII.

HENSING. In Alb. Halleri Disput. Anatom. selectæ, vol. i. Diss. inaug., De Peritoneo. Gissæ, 1724, XXIII.

HESSELBACH. Lehre von den Eingeweidebrüchen, Bd. I. Würzburg, 1829.
HIS. Anatomie Menschel. Embryonen, III., 1885.
HUGHES, A. Guy's Hospital Report, Series III., vol. ii., 1856.
HUSCHKE. Lehre von den Eingeweiden und Sinnesorganen des Menschel. Körpers. Leipzig, 1844.
HUNTINGTON, G. S. Studies in the Development of the Alimentary Canal, I. Medical Report of the Society of the Lying-in Hospital. New York, 1893.
HARMAN, N. BISHOP. Journal of Anatomy and Physiology, vol. xxxii., p. 665. The Duodeno-Jejunal Flexure: its Variations and their Significance.

JOMINI. Revue Médicale de la Suisse Romande, 2 année, 1882 (xvi. année du Bulletin de la Société Medicale de la Suisse Romande).
JONNESCO. 1. Anatomie topographique du Duodénum et Hernies Duodénales. Paris, Legrosnier et Babé, 1889.
2. Hernies int. Retro-Peritoneales. Paris, 1890. G. Steinheil.
3. Poirier's Traité d'Anatomie humaine, vol. iv.

KLEBS. Handbuch der Pathol. Anat., Bd. I. Berlin, 1869.
KLOB. Hernia Retro-Peritonealis. Wochenblatt der Zeitschrift der K. K. Gesellschaft der Aerzte in Wien, No. 24, Jahrg. vii., Juni 12, 1861.
KRAUSS. Hernia Retro-Peritonealis Treitzii. Inaugural Dissertation. Erlangen, 1884.
KUNDRAT. Vortrag in der K. K. Gesellschaft d. Aerzte, Wien, Januar 17, 1873.
KRÖNLEIN. Archiv. für Klinische Chirurgie, 1876, 1880, and 1881.
KELYNACK, T. N. A Contribution to the Pathology of the Vermiform Appendix. London, 1893.

LAMBL. 1. Reisebericht, 1856, Italienische Vierteljahrsschrift für die pract. Heilkunde, Jahrg. xvi., 1859, Bd. I., Prag.
2. Beobachtungen und Studien aus dem Gebiete d. Path. Anat. und Histol. aus dem Franz Josef Kinder Hospital in Prag. Prag, 1860.
LANDZERT. Ueber die Hernia Retro-Peritonealis, etc. (Treitz). Beiträge z. Anat. und Histol., Heft I. St. Petersburg, 1872

LANGER. 1. Die Peritonealtaschen am Cæcum. Wochenblatt der Zeitschrift der K. K. Gesellschaft der Aerzte in Wien, No. 17, April 23, 1862.
    2. Lehrbuch der Anatomie des Menschen. Wien, 1865.

LAUTNER. Zeitschrift der K. K. Gesellschaft der Aerzte in Wien. Jahrg. i., Bd. II.

LEICHTENSTERN. Handbuch der Spec. Pathologie und Therapie, herausgegeben von Dr. H. v. Ziemssen, Bd. VII., 2 Halfte. Krankheiten des chylopoetischen Apparates, I. Leipzig, 1878. English translation.

LUSCHKA. 1. Ueber die Peritoneale Umhüllung des Blinddarms und über die Fossa ileo-cæcalis. Virchow's Archiv., Bd. XXI., 1861.
    2. Die organische Musculatur verschiedener Falten des menschlichen Bauchfells. Archiv für Anatomie und Physiologie, 1862.
    3. Anatomie d. Bauches.

LAWRENCE, SIR W. On Ruptures. Fifth edition.

LOCKWOOD, C. B. 1. Hunterian Lectures on Hernia. London, 1889.
    2. Retro-Peritoneal Hernia of the Vermiform Appendix. Pathological Society's Transactions, vol. xli., 1890, p. 118.

LOCKWOOD AND ROLLESTON. On the Fossæ round the Cæcum, etc. Journal of Anatomy and Physiology, vol. xxvi., 1892, p. 130.

LITTLE, T. E. Internal Strangulation. Anatomy of the Vermiform Appendix. Dublin Journal of Medical Science, vol. lii., 1871, p. 237.

MAJOLI. Storia di una occlusione lenta dell' Intestino cagionata dal passagio e dallo strazzamento di un' ansa del crosso attraverso il Forame del Winslow. In Rivista Clinica di Bologna, anno 1884.

MECKEL. Handbuch der Pathol. Anatomie. Leipzig, 1816. Bd. II.

MONRO. 1. Observation on Crural Hernia, to which is prefixed a General Account of the other Varieties of Hernia. Edinburgh, 1803.
    2. Medical Essays and Observations, vol. iv., Art. 2.

MORGAGNI. De sedibus et causis morborum. Epist. XLIII., Art. 14.

MOUTARD-MARTIN. Anomalie du Péritoine. Bulletin de la Société Anatomique, XLV., année 1870, 2ᵉ série, 15ᵉ vol., 1874.
MULLER. Hernia Retro-Peritonealis. Innere Darmeinklemmung, Laparotomie, Tod, Autopsie. Pesther Med. Chir. Presse, Budapest, 1881, XVII.
MACALISTER, A. On two Dissimilar Forms of Perityphlic Pouches. Proceedings of the Royal Irish Academy, July, 1875.
MOTT, F. W. Pathological Society's Transactions, vol. xl., 1889, p. 105. Hernia into Fossa Iliaco-Subfascialis.
MITCHELL, LOUIS G. Personal communication.

NEUBAUER. Descriptio anatomica rarissimi peritonæi conceptaculi tenuia intestina a reliquis abdominis visceribus seclusa tenentis. Opera anatomica collecta. Editionem curavit Georgius Conradus Hinderer, Francofurti et Lipsiæ, 1786.
NOVELLO. Nel No. 38 della Gazetta Medica delle Provincie de Venete (Annuario delle Science Mediche dell' anno 1881), anno xii. Redatto dai Dottori Schivardie Fini, e publicato in Milano nell 1882 della case Editrice Dott. H. F. Vollardi.
NEUMANN. Ein Fall von operativ geheilter Hernia Retro-Peritonealis Mesenterico-Parietalis. Deutsche Zeitschrift für Chirurgie, 1898, p. 476. Band XLVII.

PARISE. Mémoire sur Deux Variétés de Hernie. Mémoires de la Société de Chirurgie de Paris, 1858, tome ii.
PEYROT. De l'Invention Chirurgicale dans l'Occlusion Intestinale. Thèse d'aggrégation, Paris, 1880.
PYE-SMITH. On Retro-Peritoneal Hernia. Guy's Hospital Reports, Series III., vol. xvi., 1871, p. 131. Pathological Society s Transactions, 1867, p. 108. Personal communication.
PEACOCK. Mesocolic Hernia as a Cause of Intestinal Obstruction. London Journal of Medicine, October, 1849.
PARTRIDGE. Internal Strangulation of the End of the Small Intestine (Ileum), Produced by its Passage through an Aperture in the Mesentery of the Appendix Vermiformis. Pathological Society's Transactions, vol. xii., 1861, p. 110.
PERIGNON. Thèse de Paris, 1892.

RENAUT. Gazette Médicale de Paris, 1878.

RIDGE AND HILTON. Case of Strangulation of the Jejunum relieved by Gastrotomy, with Observations on the Diagnosis and Treatment of Intestinal Obstructions within the Abdomen. Read before the Hunterian Society, January 18, 1854. Reprinted from the Association Medical Journal.

RIEUX. Considérations sur l'Étranglement de l'Intestin dans la Cavité Abdominale et sur un Mode d'Étranglement non Décrit par les Auteurs. Thèse de Doctorat soutenue le 22 juin, 1853. Paris, 1853.

ROKITANSKY. Handbuch der Pathol. Anatomie. Wien, 1842, Bd. III.

ROSER. Archiv für Physiol. Heilkunde von Roser und Wunderlich, 1843.

SANDIFORT. Tabulæ Intestini Duodeni. Lugd. Bat., 1780.

SANTORINI. Tabulæ 17 Santorini. Parma, 1775.

SCHIEFFERDECKER. 1. Beiträge zur Topographie des Darms. Archiv für Anatomie und Physiologie von His und Braune, 1886.
2. Beiträge zur Topographie des Darms. Ebendaselbst, 1887.

SCHOTT. Wochenblatt der Zeitschrift der K. K. Gesellschaft der Aerzte in Wien, No. 44, October 29, 1862.

SHATTOCK. Hernia into the Fossa Duodeno-Jejunalis. Transactions of the Pathological Society of London, vol. xxxvi., 1885.

SNOW. London Medical Gazette, 1846.

SOVERINI. Novi Commentarii Academiæ Scientiarum Instituti Bononiensis, tome viii. Bononiæ, 1846.

SQUARE. A Case of Strangulated Internal Hernia into the Foramen of Winslow. The British Medical Journal, vol. i., 1886.

STAUDENMAYER. Duodeno-Jejunal Hernie mit Erscheinungen von Darmverengerung. Inaugural Dissertation vorgel. d. Tubinger Facultät. Stuttgart, 1886.

STRAZEWSKI. Médecine Russe. Journal Hebdomadaire de Médecine et d'Hygiène, Nos. 43-45. 1888.

SYMINGTON-JOHNSON. The Relations of the Peritoneum to the Descending Colon. Journal of Anatomy and Physiology, 1892, p. 530.

TARENETZKY. Beiträge zur Anatomie des Darmkanals. Mémoires de l'Académie de St. Pétersbourg, Série VII., tome xxviii., 1881.

TOLDT. 1. Bau und Wachsthumsverhältnisse der Gekröse des Menschl. Darmkanals. Denkschriften der Kais. Academie der Wissenschaften zu Wien, February, 1879. Bd. XLI.
2. Zur Charact. u. Entstehungsgesch. d. Rec. Duodeno-Jejunalis. Prager Medic. Wochenschr., 1879, No. 23.
3. Die Darmgekröse und Netze im Gesetzmäss. u. Gesetzwidr. Zustand. Denkschr. d. Kais. Akad. d. Wissensch. Math. Naturw. Klasse, Bd. LVI., 1889.

TREITZ. Hernia Retro-Peritonealis. Ein Beitrag zur Geschichte innerer Hernien. Prag, 1857.

TREVES. 1. The Anatomy of the Intestinal Canal and Peritoneum in Man. Hunterian Lectures. London, 1885.
2. Clinical Lecture on Hernia into the Foramen of Winslow. Delivered at the London Hospital. Lancet, October 13, 1888.

TUFFIER. Étude sur le Cæcum et ses Hernies. Arch. Générales de Médecine. Juin, 1887.

TUBBY, A. H. Personal communication, and British Medical Journal, vol. ii., 1898.

TURNER. Centralblatt für Chirurgie, No. 42, 1892, p. 840.

VIRCHOW, R. Historisches, Kritisches und Positives z. Lehre d. Unterleibs-Affectionen. Virchow's Archiv., Bd. V.

WAGNER. Beobachtungen und Abhandlungen aus dem Gebiete der Natur und Heilkunde. Einige Beobachtungen innerer Brüche. Med. Jahrbücher des K. K. Österreichischen Staates. A. J. Freiherr von Stift. Bd. XIII., oder neue Folge, Bd. IV. Wien, 1833.

WALDEYER. Hernia Retro-Peritonealis nebst Bemerkungen zur Anatomie des Peritoneum. Breslau, 1868, zum zweiten Male abgedruckt in Virchow's Archiv., 1874.

WIDERHOFER. Jahrbuch der Kinderh. Jahrg. ii. (s. bei Schott).

ZWAARDEMAKER. Hernia Retro-Peritonealis Incarcerata. Nederlandsh Militair Geneeskunding Archief van de Landmacht, het Oost-en-West Indish Leger. Jaargang 8^e, 1er Aflevering, 1884, Utrecht.

I.—SPECIMEN 1279. ST. THOMAS'S HOSPITAL MUSEUM.

Left Duodenal Hernia.

'A preparation showing a hernia of the jejunum about the size of an orange into the fossa duodeno-jejunalis. The colon has been raised in order to expose the small intestine, which has been filled with plaster of Paris. The mouth of the peritoneal sac is about 1 inch in diameter, and lies immediately below the termination of the duodenum, the intestine within it comprising the highest few coils of the jejunum. The contents were readily removable from the sac after death; the hernia was found accidentally in a child.'

This is the most beautiful specimen of a left duodenal hernia in the early stage that I have met with. In the margin of the orifice the inferior mesenteric vein is distinctly seen.

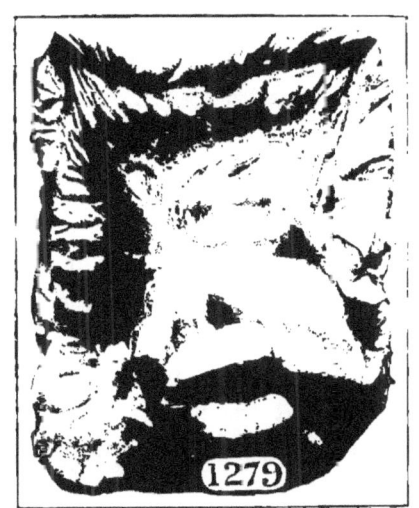

I.—ST. THOMAS'S HOSPITAL.

II.—SPECIMEN 2696 E. ROYAL COLLEGE OF SURGEONS.

LEFT DUODENAL HERNIA.

' The left end of a transverse colon, with the adjacent portion of the mesocolon seen from behind. At the root of the mesocolon is a globular peritoneal sac 5 inches in diameter, which contains almost the whole of the small intestines. The mouth of the sac, measuring 9 inches in circumference, transmits the two extremities of the included intestine. The upper one is the first part of the jejunum, and is adherent to the neck as it enters the sac, while the lower coil, which belongs to the last few inches of the ileum, leaves the sac with its mesentery, and courses behind it to reach the ileo-cæcal valve.

' Physical examination of the abdomen during life gave negative results. The patient was a woman aged sixty-nine, who died of cylindrical-celled epithelioma of the ileo-cæcal valve.'

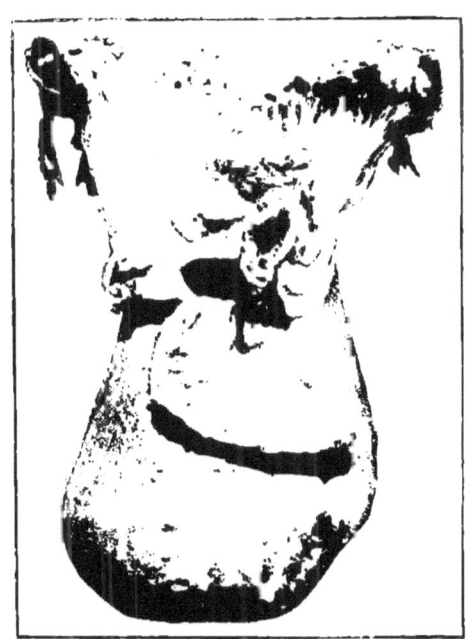

II.—ROYAL COLLEGE OF SURGEONS.

III.—SPECIMEN 1083. GUY'S HOSPITAL MUSEUM.

LEFT DUODENAL HERNIA.

'The splenic flexure and descending part of a colon in the angle between which is situated a globular peritoneal sac measuring about 4 inches in diameter, and containing several feet of small intestine. The mouth of the sac is directed towards the vertebral column, and along its anterior margin is seen the left colic artery.'

This is the specimen which was described by Dr. Pye-Smith in his paper in the Guy's Hospital Reports. The specimen was removed from a dissecting-room subject. The photograph is not a very good one, but that is the fault of the specimen. The inferior mesenteric vein is well seen in the anterior margin of the sac.

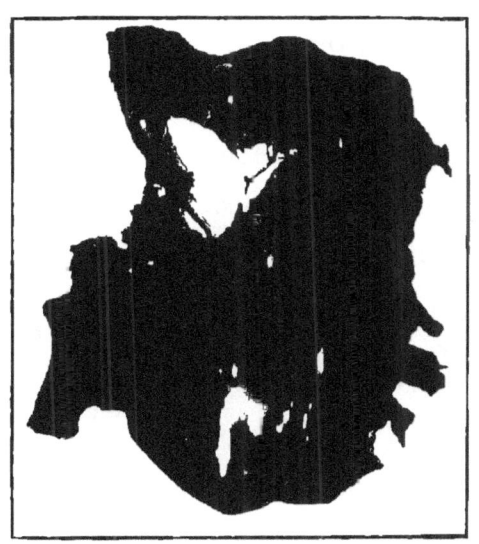

III.—SPECIMEN 1083. GUY'S HOSPITAL.

IV.—ST. MARY'S HOSPITAL MUSEUM.

Right Duodenal Hernia.

In the Pathological Society's Transactions, Mr. Jackson Clarke gives the following account:

'A man of middle age was admitted, under Mr. Page, into St. Mary's Hospital, with symptoms of acute intestinal obstruction. He said he had been seized with sudden pain, which caused him to fall down in the street. Mr. Page performed abdominal section. This revealed a large, smooth, rounded formation which had the appearance of an ordinary ovarian cystoma, but gave a tympanitic note. After passing a hand into the abdominal cavity, Mr. Page was able to withdraw the whole of the small intestine from an aperture at the lower part of the hernia. The patient gradually sank after the operation.

'Examination after death revealed a large flaccid sac lying to the left of the back part of the mesentery, and consisting of a double layer of peritoneum. Into this the whole of the small intestine could easily be replaced. After this had been done, the parts had the appearance shown in the photograph. About one foot of the upper part of the ileum was deeply congested; the rest of the small intestine had a normal appearance. The congested portion had probably been twisted within the sac. By raising the lower and left portion of the hernia upwards and to the right the arrangement of the parts at the neck of the sac could easily be seen. The aperture easily admitted the closed hand. In front it was bounded by the superior mesenteric artery, covered by peritoneum; behind by the peritoneum covering the posterior abdominal wall as it passed to form the posterior portion of the sac, ceasing at the inner edge of the ascending colon. The transverse mesocolon was present, but short, and it was attached in the usual manner. The duodeno-jejunal fossa was absent. The condition had the appearance of being congenital, and the facts might be expressed by saying that the small intestine had been rotated through 360°, first to the left, then backwards, next to the right behind the superior mesenteric vessels, and lastly forwards. The sac may be described as consisting of that part of the mesentery which lies between the superior mesenteric vessels and the attachment of the mesentery to the posterior abdominal wall. The whole of the third part of the duodenum was to the right of the superior mesenteric vessels, and possessed a short mesentery.'

Brösike states that in all cases of right duodenal hernia there must be a posterior adhesion of the upper few inches of the jejunum. In this case there is an absence rather than an excess of the normal "*physiological adhesion.*"

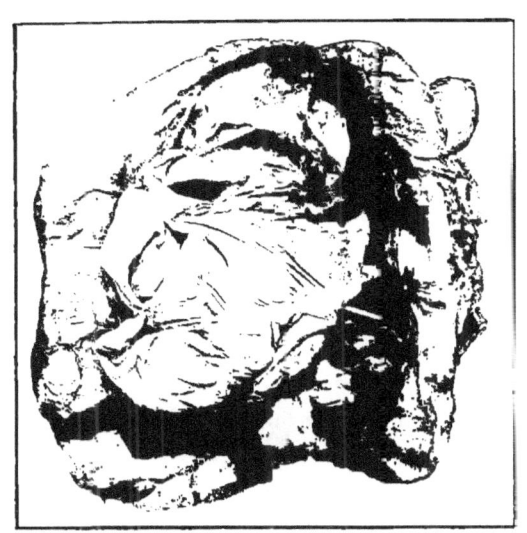

IV.—ST. MARY'S HOSPITAL.

V.—SPECIMEN 1084. GUY'S HOSPITAL MUSEUM.

Right Duodenal Hernia.

'A cæcum with the ascending and transverse colon and a coil of ileum. About 18 inches of the coil of ileum are contained in a sac formed from the peritoneum, and situated between the ascending colon and the vertebral column. The mouth of the sac is directed downwards towards the pelvis, and does not appear to have constricted the hernia.'

This is the specimen of Dr. Moxon's referred to by Dr. Pye-Smith in the concluding paragraph of his paper in the Guy's Hospital Reports. I was not sure that this was the specimen, and I therefore wrote and asked Dr. Pye-Smith to inform me. This he has very courteously done. Dr. Moxon and Dr. Pye-Smith both considered the hernia as 'subcæcal.' In the specimen, and also in the photograph, the cæcum and appendix are quite normal. In the anterior margin of the sac can be very distinctly seen the superior mesenteric artery. This is clearly an example, therefore, of right duodenal hernia.

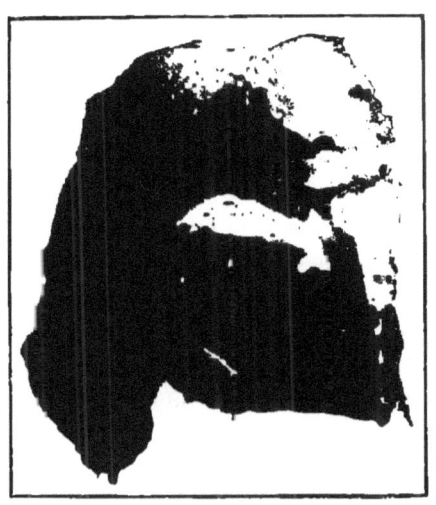

V.—SPECIMEN 1084. GUY'S HOSPITAL.

VI. A and B.

A Specimen of Right Duodenal Hernia.

A shows the normal position of the parts, the cæcum and appendix below, the ascending colon vertical. The sac, containing all the small intestines, from the duodeno-jejunal flexure to the cæcum, lies chiefly to the inner side of the colon. A distinct mesocolon is present. The sac passes behind the colon and appears on the outer side.

B shows the emptied sac. Running along the anterior margin of the orifice of the sac can be seen the superior mesenteric artery. The size of the hernial orifice is indicated by the white lines.

This specimen, a perfect one of its kind, has been preserved in the post-mortem room of the Leeds General Infirmary by Dr. T. Wardrop Griffith.

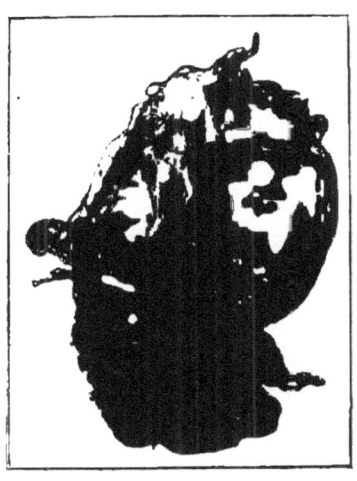

VI. A.—RIGHT DUODENAL HERNIA.

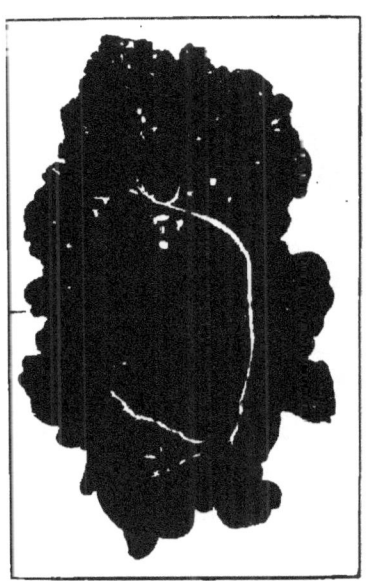

The line of superior mesenteric artery.

VI. B.—RIGHT DUODENAL HERNIA. THE SAC IS EMPTY.

VII.—SPECIMEN 1281. ST. THOMAS'S HOSPITAL.

'A cæcum, etc., with the terminal portion of the ileum. Behind the ascending colon are two capacious pouches of peritoneum, situate one immediately above the other, and freely communicating with the general peritoneal cavity on the right side. The vermiform appendix lies in the lower of the sacs.'

This is the most perfect example of two retro-colic fossæ, external and internal, that I have seen. The specimen shows even better than the photograph.

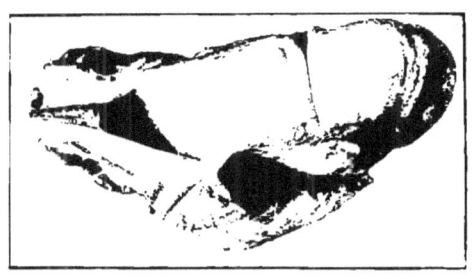

VII.—SPECIMEN 1281. ST. THOMAS'S HOSPITAL.

VIII.

A RETRO-COLIC HERNIA OF THE VERMIFORM APPENDIX.

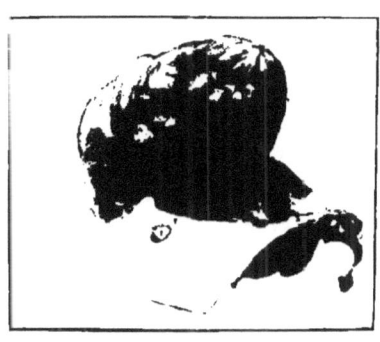

VIII.—THE RETRO-COLIC FOSSA, CONTAINING THE VERMIFORM APPENDIX.

IX.—ST. BARTHOLOMEW'S HOSPITAL.

Intersigmoid Hernia.

The specimen shows the intersigmoid fossa, the cæcum, and colon. It is taken from Mr. Eve's case of hernia, described fully in the text. The diagram there given and the photograph should be compared.

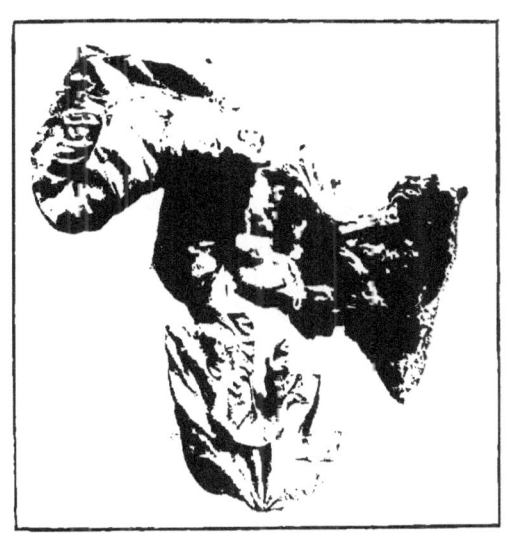

IX.—ST. BARTHOLOMEW'S HOSPITAL

X.

Female child, aged thirteen months. Death from catarrhal pneumonia, following measles.

On opening the abdomen, it was found that the greater part of the ascending colon was covered behind by peritoneum, so as to lie between the two layers of the mesentery. To the left of the abdominal cavity a sac containing bowel was seen. This sac was about 4½ inches long, and 3½ inches in the transverse diameter, and extended from the middle line, where the entrance was placed, to the outer side of the descending colon. A short descending mesocolon was present. In the vertical direction the sac reached from the pancreas to a little below the brim of the pelvis. The sac contained rather more than half the intestine. On removing the bowel from the sac, three small descending intussusceptions were seen. The orifice of the sac, which looked directly to the right, admitted four fingers. The edge was very sharp, and contained the inferior mesenteric vein and the ascending branch of the left colic artery. The duodeno-jejunal flexure lies in the sac at the upper and inner extremity. [For explanation of this condition, see the text, p. 49.] The inferior duodenal fold is present, though small, and not as acutely defined as it generally is in children.

No symptoms were present during life.

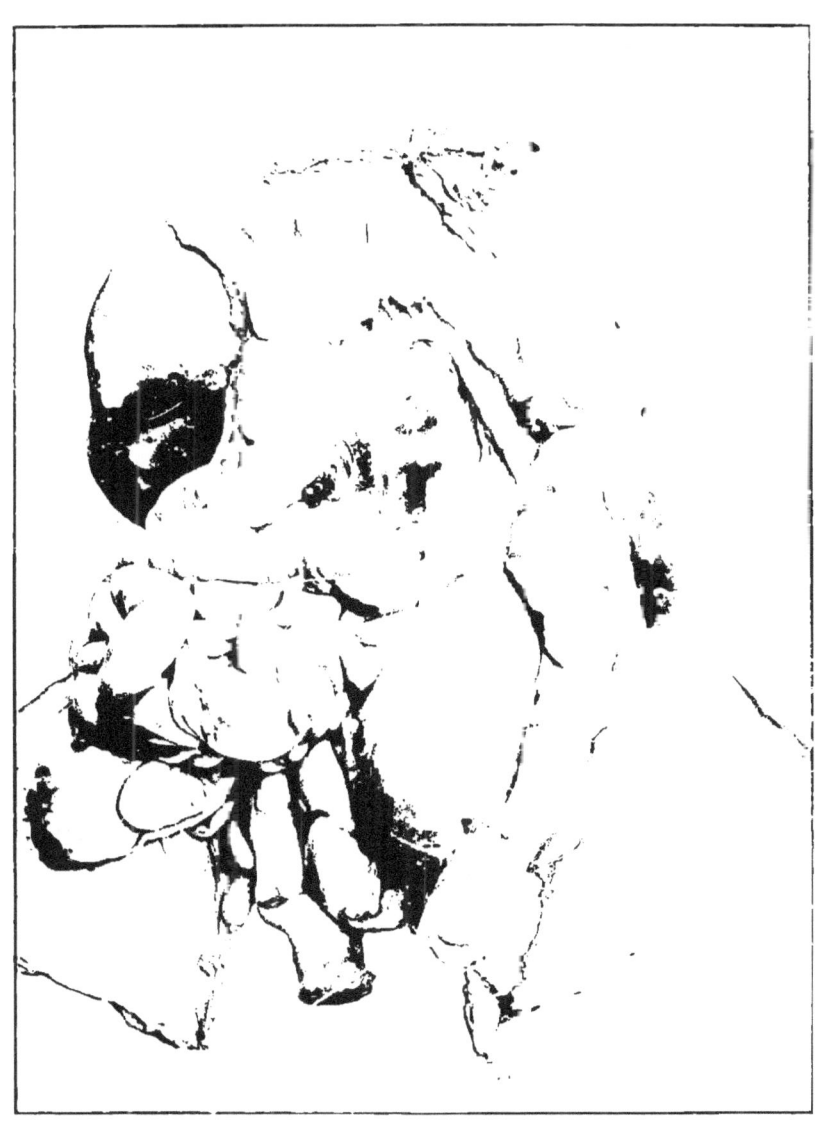

X.—LEFT DUODENAL HERNIA. DR. GRIFFITHS' CASE.

XI. AND XII.

These two photographs have been sent to me by Dr. Louis Mitchell, of Chicago, just in time for insertion in this volume. I must express my warmest thanks to Dr. Mitchell for his courtesy. The description of the case is given in the text on pp. 55 and 56.

XI.—Showing sac as it appeared on opening the abdomen.

XII.—Showing sac and contents lifted up, with slip of paper under the ileum as it left the sac.

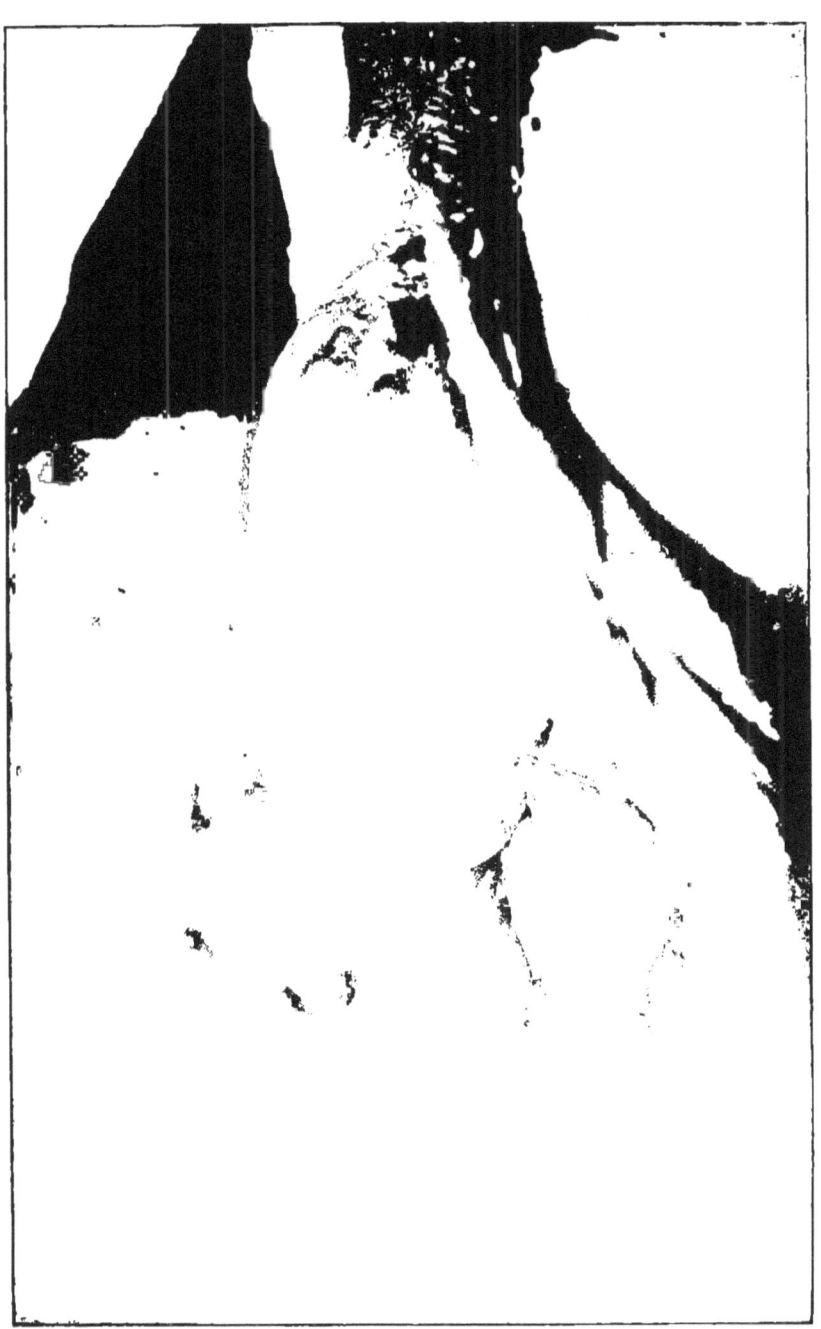

XL.—SHOWING SAC AS IT APPEARED ON OPENING ABDOMEN.

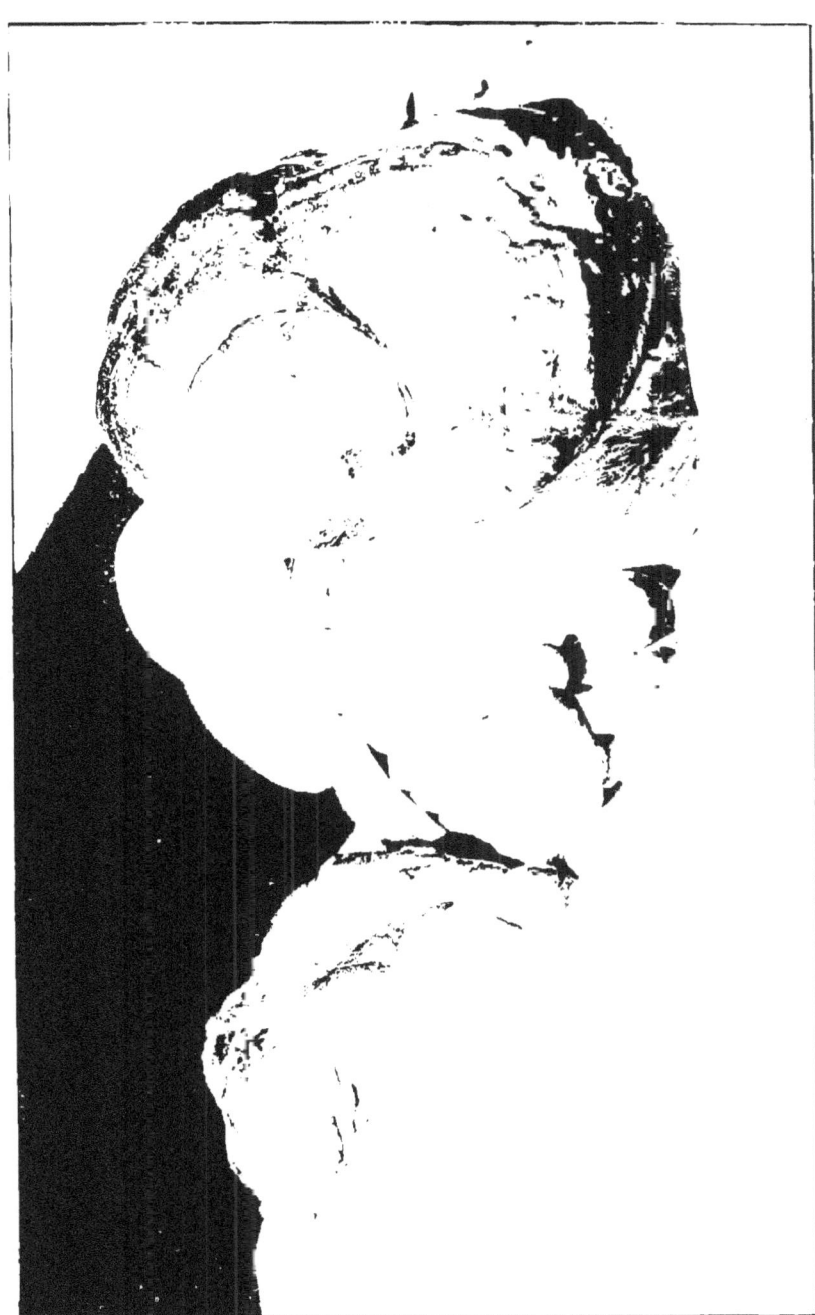

XII. SHOWING SAC AND CONTENTS LIFTED UP, WITH STAKE PASSED UNDER ILEUM AS IT LEFT SAC

www.ingramcontent.com/pod-product-compliance
Lightning Source LLC
Chambersburg PA
CBHW020259170426
43202CB00008B/436